Small Remedies &
Interesting Cases VI

PROCEEDINGS OF THE 1994 PROFESSIONAL CASE CONFERENCE

Editors: Stephen King, ND, DHANP
Sheryl Kipnis, ND, DHANP
Cathie Scott

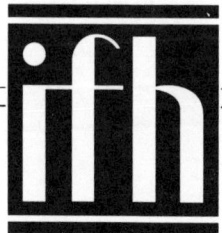

International
Foundation
for
Homeopathy

INTERNATIONAL FOUNDATION FOR HOMEOPATHY

The IFH is a nonprofit organization with over 2,500 lay and professional members around the world. It is dedicated to promoting public awareness of classical homeopathy and to maintaining the highest standards of homeopathic practice and education. The foundation accomplishes these goals by holding public and professional courses, conducting research, promoting the establishment of homeopathic medical schools, and publishing *Resonance*, a bimonthly magazine for its members.

OFFICE

2366 Eastlake Avenue East, Suite 325, Seattle, WA 98102 • (206) 324-8230

ACKNOWLEDGEMENTS

Thanks to Kathy Fogarty for transcribing the proceedings of this conference, to Edie Neeson for proofreading assistance, and to Anne Walton Design and Lillian Sugahara for graphic design and typesetting.

Drs. King and Kipnis also thank co-editor Cathie Scott for her many hours of editorial work in helping to give this book its final form.

And, as always, we especially thank the conference speakers for sharing from their clinical experience. Each of you has added to our common body of knowledge.

WITH GRATEFUL THANKS

A portion of the editorial and printing costs of this publication was underwritten by a generous donation from Standard Homeopathic Company. Jack Craig and the folks at Standard Homeopathic have provided support for each of the six IFH case conference proceedings.

On behalf of all homeopathic practitioners and patients, and for all others who will benefit from the information preserved here, the IFH extends special thanks for your kind assistance.

TABLE OF CONTENTS

PREFACE .... *vii*

THREE CASES OF MENORRHAGIA
  Judyth Reichenberg-Ullman, ND, DHANP, MSW 1

THREE CASES OF INFERTILITY AND
  PELVIC INFLAMMATORY DISEASE (PID)
  David Riley, MD 35

CLINICAL EXPERIENCES WITH CARCINOSIN
  Ahmed Currim, MD, PhD 67

HOMEOPATHY: WORKING IN THE SACRED SPACE
  Karl Robinson, MD 101

A HOMEOPATHIC SOJOURN IN INDIA
  Nancy Herrick, PA-C 125

THREE PALLADIUM CASES: EXPLORING THE ESSENTIAL ELEMENTS
  Roger Morrison, MD 151

TWO CASES OF OBSESSIVE-COMPULSIVE DISORDER
  Valerie Ohanian, AHCH 171

A CASE OF DEPRESSION AND LOSS OF JOY
  Anne Schadde, Heilprakterin 199

A SMALL BUT USEFUL REMEDY
  Sheryl Kipnis, ND, DHANP, and Stephen King, ND, DHANP 223

A CASE OF PARANOID SCHIZOPHRENIA
  Steven Olsen, ND, DHANP 263

COMPUTER-ASSISTED ANALYSIS IN DIFFICULT CASES
  Guy Kokelenberg, MD, and Roger van Zandvoort 291

SACCHARUM OFFICINALE, THE MAGIC SUGAR!
  Tinus Smits, MD 335

PREFACE

One of the nicest things about the 1994 IFH Professional Case Conference (the sixth annual) was the presence and contribution of more homeopaths from around the world—from Europe, the United Kingdom, and Australia.

As Guy Kokelenberg of Belgium said, "It is nice to travel halfway around the world and realize we are using the same homeopathic language. It feels like coming home to family." The North American branch of the homeopathic family hopes that you will return for next year's conference and bring even more of your colleagues with you!

Three other things were noteworthy. First, there were cases that used remedies, such as Scorpion and Hydrogen, that were recently proved by Jeremy Sherr and others. We are all in your debt.

Second, the growing influence of the ideas of Rajan Sankaran of India—the latest "wave" in homeopathy—was quite apparent. Several speakers and audience members made reference to Sankaran's teaching, which has expanded our ability to practice effectively.

Third, the presentations and discussions at this year's conference seemed to reflect a broader, perhaps a more spiritually based approach to practice. It was evident that our community continues to explore the interface between the art and the science of homeopathic medicine.

These published proceedings once again reflect our commitment to preserve this information for all present and future homeopaths.

Perhaps a word about the notations used in the cases would be helpful for some readers. While taking cases, homeopaths often underline symptoms for emphasis. A given symptom may be underlined zero, one, two, or three times, depending on the intensity, clarity, and spontaneity of the symptom as given by the patient. The strongest emphasis is represented by a symptom underlined three times.

In this book the underlining is given as a number in parentheses after the symptom. Thus, "irritable in the morning on waking (3)" means that the homeopath felt this was a strong symptom in the patient's case and therefore underlined it three times for emphasis. If no number follows a particular symptom, then the symptom was not underlined by the homeopath.

The response around the world to the five previous proceedings published by the IFH has been both enthusiastic and gratifying. May each prescriber's ability to help those in need be increased by the contents of this book.

Sheryl Kipnis, ND, DHANP
Stephen King, ND, DHANP

IFH
Professional Course
in Homeopathy

ABOUT THE COURSE

The purpose of the IFH Professional Course is to provide thorough instruction in classical homeopathy to those health professionals who seek to undertake the serious study of homeopathy. It is an in-depth, comprehensive course that will allow the participant to become truly proficient in classical homeopathy.

In order to enable busy practitioners to attend, the IFH Professional Course consists of two levels, each a 120-hour intensive module (one weekend per month over five months). The first module, Level I, is for the beginning student who has little prior training or experience in homeopathy. Level II is for the intermediate student who has completed Level I or is admitted by permission. Each "weekend" session meets Thursday through Sunday. This format enables the student to fully digest and use the knowledge and experience of each session before going on to more advanced material.

The course is open to licensed health care practitioners, i.e.: MD, DO, ND, DC, acupuncturist, DDS, DVM, RN, PA, RPH, etc. For further information contact the IFH.

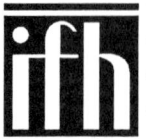

International Foundation for Homeopathy
2366 Eastlake Avenue East Suite #325
Seattle WA 98102-3366 ◆ 206-324-8230
"We train homeopaths."

Judyth Reichenberg-Ullman,
ND, DHANP, MSW

THREE CASES
OF
MENORRHAGIA

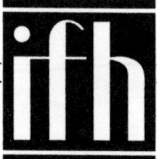

Judyth Reichenberg-Ullman graduated in 1983 from Bastyr College of Naturopathic Medicine and has been practicing homeopathy ever since. She completed the IFH Professional Course in 1985 and has taken Paul Herscu's course through the New England School of Homeopathy. Judyth is a diplomate and past vice president of the Homeopathic Academy of Naturopathic Physicians. She also is president of the IFH board of directors and is an instructor in the IFH Professional Course. Judyth writes extensively for Resonance, The Townsend Letter for Doctors, EastWest Natural Health, *and other publications. She specializes in women's health care, and practices in Seattle with her husband, Robert Ullman, ND (also an IFH instructor and board member). Judyth and Robert recently studied with Rajan Sankaran in India.*

Introduction: A Short Acute Case

The more I study homeopathy, the more I am overwhelmed by how much there is to learn. I am still somewhat amazed and grateful when I get the prescription right!

By way of introduction, let's begin with a quick acute case that I saw two weeks ago. It is a case I found quite interesting. The patient was a nine-year-old girl. She did not actually have an appointment scheduled with me. The family had brought two other daughters for first office calls, and her mother simply mentioned at the beginning that this third daughter also had a problem. The mother wondered if there might be a few minutes at the end when I could do something for her. They had driven quite a distance, and I agreed to see the girl if there was time after the other visits.

When the girl walked into my office, she had an enlarged left submandibular gland approximately the size of a tennis ball! I said, "This is what I am supposed to spend a few minutes on at the end of the other visits?" Something obviously needed to be done.

About eight weeks earlier, the girl felt some pain on the left side of her jaw. Two weeks later, she developed this left submandibular swelling. In addition to being about the size of a tennis ball, it was rock hard and rather red. She said the redness occurred from having bumped into something.

So, she had the swelling and some pain radiating to the left ear. That was essentially the case. I could find nothing else of significance. Are there any quick ideas about a prescription?

Suzanne Adams: I thought of Bromium, for the left-sided, rock-hard glandular swelling.

Reichenberg-Ullman: Yes, that is just how I thought about it.

I was naturally quite concerned about the girl. The family thought that she probably had mumps. I questioned that diagnosis. I thought perhaps she had a salivary tumor, or even possibly Hodgkin's disease. I gave Bromium 1M, a single dose, and instructed the mother to take the girl to a pediatrician in their town if there was no improvement within two or three days.

The mother called me five days later and said that the swelling was considerably reduced and that there was now some itching in the area. With this improvement as feedback, I advised her to wait and keep me informed. I talked to the mother just yesterday. She reported that the swelling had completely gone and that the girl was doing fine in general. So, this was an interesting case that was a little frightening for me at the time.

Now let's look at the three cases I brought to share with you today.

[Editors' Note: Dr. Reichenberg's spontaneous comments, made while presenting the cases, are bracketed and italicized.]

Case Number 1

Female
Age 42

Initial Visit: March 20, 1992

(Video excerpts were shown.)

I've had a series of head colds since Christmas. Recent sinusitis. Took Amoxycillin for one week. Developed a rash. Benadryl was prescribed. Got anaphylaxis from the Benadryl. Then took prednisone for several days. The episode really scared me.

I've had heavy periods (3) in the past three years. They start every 32 days and last five days. The flow is getting heavier and heavier (3). The first day I use a combination of tampons and pads, which I change every 1½ hours. Clots (2). No pain. Diarrhea the first 24 to 48 hours (2). Bright red, medium-sized clots (2); bright red flow (2). Slight spotting mid-cycle.

I have three daughters. My pregnancies were fine except for high blood pressure when I was pregnant with twins.

My sexual energy has been down to zero for a long time (3). I'm getting a divorce. I can hardly wait to get it over with. My marriage has been really hard the past four years. I want more contact. He's really private. That's been hard on the kids, which is hard on me.

I am ready to fall asleep any time, any place (3). I wake at 2:30 or 3:00 a.m. most nights (2) and stew (2). I toss and turn for two hours (2). I fantasize about hiding under the bed for six months, waking up, and having it (the divorce) be all over.

For the 21 years I was married I slept on my left side. Now that I'm alone, I sleep on my right side.

Lots of moles on my skin.

When I am with my spirit group, I bleed really heavily for two days. [*She is involved in a Native American tradition.*] It's as if my whole pelvis has opened and relaxed, as if I'm a river.

I bled heavily for two weeks after both pregnancies and after my wisdom tooth surgery.

Chilly (2). I like lots of blankets at night and the window open.

I like bread (3), avocados (2), milk (2), and salt (2).

I don't like beer (2), coffee (2), and spicy food (2).

Thirsty for icy cold drinks (3).

I'm secretive (2), private (2). I'm open and friendly in relationships, but don't want people to get too close to me. Affectionate. I withdraw before my feelings are hurt (2).

Afraid of flying (3). I'm afraid that I can't get away (3). I plan escape routes when I'm on planes or ferries (3). Also afraid of heights (1) and water (2).

I have difficulty saying what I want (2). I ruminate and ruminate, collect information, and never make a decision (2). There's always one more piece of information. I'm never ready to take action.

My father died in 1987. I haven't seen my mother for seven months. She's deteriorating rapidly.

I was very depressed after my father's death. I cried, but only in private because it would make me appear needy. I've been shut down to myself (2). To really feel my emotions gets in the way of functioning. "Let's be practical."

I was spoiled as a child. I was the only daughter. Three brothers. I was very, very good.

[*Looking at the video of this case and the two cases that follow, I see that I would take the cases differently now than I did back then. After having spent time studying with Jeremy Sherr and Rajan Sankaran, I have learned to be more silent in the interview—to talk less and to interfere less.*]

> **Jim Hill:** *My first impression is that this seems like a Natrum muriaticum case, although there is a bit of Pulsatilla there, not wanting to show her feelings. Natrum muriaticum is emotionally labile, very unstable.*

Assessment: She has painless metrorrhagia and she wakes after 2 a.m. I repertorized using these two symptoms, plus FEMALE, Metrorrhagia, bright red, and MIND, Irresolution, indecision. The remedies that came up were Calcarea carbonica, Ipecacuanha, Phosphorus, Kali carbonicum, Kali ferrocyanatum, and Hamamelis.

Plan: 1. Kali ferrocyanatum 30c, single dose.
2. Call after her next period.

Follow-Up on Case Number 1

July 3, 1992

The remedy worked great. I recently discovered a cyst on my right breast. I had an ultrasound today. The diagnosis is fibrocystic breast disease.

I've been so wired for the past six months, with the divorce. It's like my body is falling apart (2).

After the remedy my period was lighter and without clots. I needed a new pad only every two hours the last time. The time before, I changed only every three hours and the pad wasn't saturated.

[*This improvement was during a time of extreme stress for her. She and her husband were in the process of divorce. They were trying to figure out how to be civil with each other and, in addition, how to manage their three children.*]

No more diarrhea with my period.

I have a huge amount of sexual energy.

I moved out of my house.

I'm no longer waking at 2:30 or 3:00 a.m. I sleep through the night.

I'd like to unzip my body and step out of it for a while (3).

I'm not chilly. In fact, I want lots of windows open all the time (3). I've always liked windows open. I also like the covers off (2).

I want fruit (2). I'm really thirsty for fruit (2). I used to get diarrhea from fruit. Not anymore.

I have less of a desire for bread, salt, and milk.

I still like cold drinks (2).

People say I look flushed.

I'm sleeping on my left side.

Assessment: The remedy is correct.

Plan: 1. Wait.
     2. Take multivitamins, multiminerals, calcium, and magnesium.
     3. Take a bike ride every evening.
     4. Decrease caffeine intake.
     5. Return in five weeks.

August 4, 1992

My periods are getting closer together and starting to get heavier. I had periods on June 19, July 11, and August 4. Each period is increasingly heavy (2). They're still painless. I had some small clots with my last period.

The divorce has finally caught up with me. I have a sensation of sinking into a hole—blackness (3).

I'm waking in the night again at 2:30 or 3:00 a.m., like before the remedy.

Less breast tenderness this time. The cysts are still there, but not as painful.

I'm really thirsty for ice water (3), especially during the past week.

Assessment: Partial relapse.

Plan: 1. Kali ferrocyanatum 200c, single dose.
     2. Return in two months.

October 27, 1992

My daughter is bulimic. She weighs 117 pounds.

My period was heavy last week with lots of clots. I didn't have diarrhea this period.

I'm not waking in the middle of the night. I'm dreaming a lot and remembering. Dreams about driving to the edge of cliffs and having to be careful not to fall off.

I'm not feeling a sense of sinking into blackness. It's more a sense of being supported in space. I have to get rid of the shell—a stripping away.

I'm still really thirsty for cold water (3), ice cold (3). I buy water in big jugs.

I like to eat rice (3) and bread (3).

I'm cold (3). Use three blankets and a down comforter.

This week I'm marginal because of my daughter.

Up until last week I felt a sense of being more even most of the time. When I do have a high or low, I return to normal within minutes.

My mind feels empty.

Assessment: Partial relapse due to stress of bulimic daughter.

Plan: 1. Kali ferrocyanatum 200c, single dose.
          2. Return in two months.

July 6, 1993

I'm doing much better.

I'm sleeping really well.

My periods have been very easy to cope with. I had a four-day period on June 24 and another started again July 4. Not heavy. It's the first time that happened.

From March through May I had some night sweats. I'd wake dripping in rivulets.

The remedy's still working.

My husband and I separated. My divorce is in progress.

My daughter has been in and out of the hospital with bulimia. Now she's doing much better.

I was evaluated for a complicated breast cyst that showed up on an ultrasound. I had a basal cell carcinoma removed from my scalp two months ago.

I'm in a new relationship.

I just feel better. I feel more in my body. Living closer to my skin. Healthier and stronger.

I'm moving to be with the kids half of each week.

My relationship is wonderful. It's like coming home. I feel like I can say anything.

I have a feeling of just dripping from the walls. I cry a lot more easily, but it feels okay. It's more like tears of gratitude. I just excuse myself and cry.

I'm doing a lot of meditating.

I sleep really well.

If anything, I'm a little warmer.

I like honeydew melon (2) and bread (3).

I feel like I've been through the tight spot in the birth canal.

Assessment: Much better.

Plan: 1. Wait.
        2. Return in six months or as needed.

March 17, 1994

It has been 17 months since I prescribed the last dose of the remedy. Since then I learned more about the remedy but I felt I still didn't understand her state as well as I could. So, in this follow-up I tried to understand her more deeply.

My periods are heavy again. I bled heavily on New Year's Eve. My hematocrit was down to 28. Now it's back to 33. I bleed really heavily when I have no breast tenderness or cramping (2).

My partner and I bought a house. My mother died one month ago. She'd been in a nursing home for a year. She no longer recognized me. There's a sense of the ceiling being gone over the top of my head, like I can grow taller. A vacuous space.

I had a recurring, scary dream about my daughter when she was a toddler. She was in diapers, 18 months old. She was drowning—in a bathtub or kiddie pool—because I wasn't paying attention. [*Note the dreams of falling into water and her feeling as if she committed a crime. These are both Ferrum symptoms.*]

What's been hardest for me is trying to get away, to make some space, to have control over some time and space. I've felt like people can reach inside me and take stuff out, like from my belly. That's where my life force is. My parents could reach inside me.

My mother was over 40 when I was born, and my father was in his mid 40s. My next oldest brother was 12. I had three siblings. I think I was too much. They wanted me to sit down and be quiet. That energy could be stolen from me because it was too much. It was as if my energy or life force was too much and had to be contained. The only place it could be let out was in private.

I was too loud and inappropriate for my father. He loved me when I was ladylike and behaved. My mother was alcoholic and wasn't there. She was profoundly depressed.

I was a very good child. My community had a fair in the summer with rides. We had a dunk tank to raise money for charity. I went in the dunk tank, and my father was livid. He was mortified because I had made a spectacle of myself in public. He wanted me to be ladylike and proud. No one ever argued with my father. He could make you feel very small.

My father died in 1986. Since then, I've been setting down that idea that I had to be a certain way. It was for my father that I stayed married as long as I did. I married at age 20. When I went back to school at 33, he said it would be my fault if the marriage failed because I wasn't at home. I had a sense of having to tone my being.

Assessment: Relapse.

Plan: 1. Kali ferrocyanatum 200c, single dose.
2. Return in four months.

Case Number 2

Female
Age 49

(Video excerpts were shown.)

Initial Visit: October 2, 1992

I'm an actress. I also do bookkeeping. I'm working right now as a weekend cashier.

My last doctor's visit was eight years ago when I tried out to be Pluto at Disneyland. I was told that I was in excellent health except for uterine fibroids.

I've never had medical insurance.

I've gained 50 pounds over the past eight years (weepy throughout most of the interview). I'm not photogenic at this size.

I'm a crier (3).

My periods have been like clockwork for years. They start at 7:30 every fourth Monday.

Several years ago I started to have a huge outpouring of blood. I have an incredibly heavy flow the first day of my period (3). I've ruined a lot of clothes. I have small clots—dark red blood the first day, then a lighter color the second day.

There's no pain. I've had 17 cramps in my entire life.

I don't have hot flashes. I have hot half hours. My cheeks get bright red (3). It's been this way for the past six years. It's totally tied to stress. I made a conscious choice not to have problems around menopause.

I get a heat rash under both breasts (1).

I have almost a constant vaginal discharge (2). It's usually white (2). I've had it for years.

I've had two marriages and a half-dozen affairs. My second marriage ended in 1983. I'm not intimate with men. I push them away because I feel unattractive (2). I want a relationship only about six times a year.

I started acting four years ago.

I have a 24-year-old daughter and a 20-year-old son. I loved mothering. I wore high heels and colored in coloring books. They loved me. I got divorced from their father when they were three and seven. The kids went to live with their dad when they were 12 and 16.

I weigh 205 pounds. I eat what I want. I know that I have to create a different attitude toward food. I nurture myself with food (crying).

I wasn't allowed to cry as a child. I usually cry about happy things.

I'm afraid of finding out that there is something very wrong with me physically or finding out that I'm out of control.

I was abused as a child. My mother was physically abusive. I thought she was trying to kill me. When I cried, she'd put her hands over my mouth and my nose. I'd pass out. I learned to stop crying very early.

I was raised a Catholic. I was never allowed to express negative feelings. I was always a good little girl and funny as shit. I think I was sexually abused very young. I think my weight is a symptom of that.

I'm a chameleon. Last winter I didn't turn the heat on at all. But heat doesn't bother me. I think I'm from another planet. I adapt.

My sleep is great. It was my escape as a child. I sleep on my side or my back (crying).

I have low back pain all the time (3). It's very hard to get out of bed in the morning. It's painful (2) and stiff (2).

I was a heavy-duty bowler at age 20. I was in three leagues. By the end of the game, I could barely stand up.

I have really strange hours. I don't have set mealtimes or rest times. I take naps. It's my middle-age rebellion.

I'm here in Seattle to get my experience behind me for acting.

I've never met a food I didn't like. I'm absolutely addicted to chocolate (3), coffee (3), caffeine (3), meat and potatoes (3), sandwiches (3), 14 different kinds of lunch meats (3), cheese and crackers (3), and salty foods (2). I must have a hamburger now and then. I like peanut butter with lots of jelly on Wonder Bread two times a year.

[*Some of Sankaran's recent teaching on case analysis has focused on categorizing the patient in terms of the mineral, plant, and animal kingdoms as another tool for determining what remedy is indicated.* (Editors' Note: See Nancy Herrick's presentation later in this book for a detailed discussion of this topic.) *She expresses her sense of humor when she says, "I want a relationship six times a year; I've had 17 cramps in my life; I like peanut butter with jelly on bread two times a year." But these statements also are examples of the "structure" that Sankaran says characterizes the language of patients needing a remedy from the mineral kingdom. This woman is quite emotional and sensitive, but there is a quality of "structure" that comes through in her manner of expression.*]

For the past ten years, fried foods haven't agreed with me (2). My body responds with gas (2), bloating (2), and sluggishness (2). I must have eaten 10,000 hamburgers at the Butter Bun when I was a teenager. The hamburgers were cooked in butter with a big pat of butter underneath, fried onions (in butter), and a buttered bun.

I'm not really thirsty, but I do like water.

I had a tubal ligation in 1974.

I was divorced in 1975.

My father died of stomach cancer at age 52 in 1965. He was an asbestos worker. His brother died of lung cancer. He also worked with asbestos.

In the past year I've been getting headaches. It feels like there's a band around my head (2). Pressing (2).

Dandruff (3).

Postnasal drip (2) my whole life.

I get a squeezing sensation in the center of my chest (2), more on the right side, about two times a month. I think it's stress.

I have a cast-iron stomach. It's a curse.

I gained 12 pounds when I was pregnant with my daughter and 9,000 pounds with my son and never lost it. My husband told me that if I had twins he wouldn't be there when I came home from the hospital.

I hated my first husband, but I had low self-esteem and was afraid to be an old maid. I made all of the decisions. My second husband was a dear friend for many years. I still love him. He didn't grow with me. He wanted to control me.

I've always been borderline anemic. My nails turn blue when I'm cold (2).

I'm a very serene person.

I wanted the whole world to like me for 45 years. I became the class clown, but I was hiding a lot of pain.

I used to be very nervous. I wanted everything to be right. I was always on edge when I was younger. I feared someone would find out I wasn't perfect.

I'm afraid of being alone (2), even though I know I've made that choice. I don't like edges (2).

My cheeks get red from exertion. In aerobics, I thought I'd have a heart attack. Normally, my cheeks are totally white.

Acting is the most important thing in my life (3).

I love eggs (3). I can't stand loud TV. I want to kill people for their loud car radios (3).

My feet get cold fast. I wear socks to bed.

I have heart palpitations when I exert.

Assessment: Uterine fibroids, menorrhagia, and back pain. I based my prescription on the painless menorrhagia, plethoric constitution, bright red or white cheeks, desire for meat, headaches, history of anemia, sensitivity to noise, and the rubric, MIND, Mirth, hilarity, and liveliness.

Plan: 1. Kali ferrocyanatum 200c, single dose.

2. Get a physical examination, including a Pap smear, pelvic ultrasound, general blood chemistries (SMAC), and mammogram.
3. Dietary recommendations.
4. Return in two months.

Follow-Up on Case Number 2

October 9, 1992

Her physical examination was unremarkable.

Laboratory results:
- Pap Class II.
- Benign cellular changes—reactive/repair.

November 25, 1992

My periods are like they were in the old days again. They last three to four days. The flow is much gentler and shorter. I can clearly say "Yes, this is a period."

My back is much better.

I'm amazed that I don't need coffee.

I've lost nine pounds. My goal is to lose five pounds each month.

My vaginal discharge is reduced. The entire female organ thing is like when I was younger.

No headaches. I haven't even noticed them.

My dandruff is still pretty bad (3).

No squeezing sensation in the center of my chest.

Assessment: Much better. Slight cervical cell changes.

Plan: 1. Wait.
       2. Take beta carotene 50,000 IU per day and folic acid 5 mg three times a day.
       3. Get another Pap smear.
       4. Return in 2½ months.

February 16, 1993

Still doing well.

No abnormal bleeding.

My back is very good, for my back.

My energy is very good.

Have kept off the nine pounds.

No headaches.

Still some chest pain when I'm stressed, but not as intense.

Physical Examination:
- Bimanual exam within normal limits.
- Pap smear repeated. (Results came back within normal limits.)

Assessment: Doing well.

Plan: 1. Wait.
       2. Return in three months.

March 29, 1993

(Six months after the original dose.)

Being in a male acting role has made me get in touch with my male side. As a girl, I was always told I was too big, like a boy.

My back still hurts.

None of my other symptoms are back.

Last week I did a lot of walking, helped a friend move. My back got progressively worse for three days, but it is better today. My back pain is like before the remedy. It was much better after I took the remedy. Lower sacral pain (2). Worse when sitting after standing (3), changing positions (2).

I just finished a normal period. I have one hot flash a week. Slight vaginal discharge before and after my period.

No more squeezing sensation in my right chest.

No headaches.

Feel good mentally and emotionally.

Food is my crutch. Now I have sweets every two or three days. Before, I had to have them every day.

Assessment: Slight relapse.

Plan: 1. Kali ferrocyanatum 30c, single dose.
          2. Call me in a few days.

April 1, 1993

Telephone consultation.

Remedy is slowly working.

June 21, 1993

This is my 50th birthday. I realize I've dreaded birthdays all my life.

The last dose of the remedy didn't really take anything away.

The bleeding is starting again, but my periods are not heavy. They change all the time (3). Irregular (3). Still painless.

Vaginal discharge again (2). Was much better after the first dose of the remedy.

My back is really bad (3). I'm stiff in the morning again (2).

The squeezing sensation in my chest has been worse lately (2), since the remedy stopped working.

I want bagels (3) and cheese (3).

I'm not in a show now. I miss the whole atmosphere.

Assessment: Relapse. The Kali ferrocyanatum 30c didn't act.

Plan: 1. Kali ferrocyanatum 200c, single dose.
2. SMAC as soon as she can afford it.

July 29, 1993

SMAC was normal, except the LDLs were slightly elevated and the cholesterol/ HDL ratio was 5.4 (normal is 4.4 or less).

Pelvic ultrasound: Seven uterine fibroids, largest measuring 4.4 by 3.7 cm. Ovaries appear normal.

September 29, 1993

My back is starting to get bad again (2). It's hard to stand up after sitting at a computer or when I get up in the morning (3). The remedy has taken care of it in the past. The pain shoots down from my lower back to left thigh (2).

I haven't lost another ounce, but that's okay. I need to make a commitment to lose weight.

I started a new job. I want to dress better. Lost three pounds since Monday.

Just got into a show. I play a bag lady.

Heavy bleeding again during periods (2). Lots of vaginal mucus in between (2).

I do have a very slight squeezing sensation in my chest.

Everything seems complete except that I don't have a relationship with a man.

Assessment: Relapse. (Last dose acted for three months.)

Plan: Kali ferrocyanatum 1M, single dose.

December 20, 1993

Received a letter from her.

I took the last remedy. It didn't have much effect for nearly a week. I was somewhat concerned but trusted somehow that it was just slower. And, for some unknown reason, that's just what happened. Slowly, one by one, the headaches, chest pain, back discomfort, and vaginal discharge became less and less. And life was easier.

(Doesn't feel she needs an appointment at this time.)

March 15, 1994

I called to see how she was doing.

"Things are cool."

Assessment: Doing well.

Plan: Return as needed.

Case Number 3

Female
Age 45

(Video excerpts were shown.)

Initial Visit: November 23, 1993

I'm having extremely heavy periods (3). The clots are so large that they scare me (3).
It's very inconvenient because I'm an outside salesperson. Within one hour, I can
saturate the heaviest pad and tampon (3). The large clots push out the tampons.
Sometimes I have to change them every 20 minutes.

I had a D & C three years ago. It's gotten gradually worse since. I don't want another
D & C.

Plus, I'm self-employed and have no insurance.

I can't plan vacations because of the bleeding (3). I have to clear my schedule. I travel
down to Oregon or up to Canada.

My periods always adjust to the schedules of the periods of the women I work with.
They were every 28 days. Since last November, they've been every 23 to 24 days,
then every 27 to 28 days, then every 23 to 24 days again.

I never have cramps.

No bloating.

No PMS.

The clots are painless. They can be larger than a double chicken liver (2).

I don't believe I'm anemic. I don't feel weak.

I eat very well.

I can get very weak and faint. (Testing showed she was not hypoglycemic.)

I have been getting migraine headaches (3) since I was ten years old. I got headaches
from cigar or cigarette smoke. At age 16 the bad migraines started, the kind where
you want to die.

At age 22 I started taking birth control pills. I had excruciating headaches after I
stopped taking the pills. Then I had an abortion. So I went back on the pill for five
years until I was 27. Then I got a Copper 7 IUD.

At age 32, after my second IUD was removed, the real heavy bleeding started. I got pregnant immediately after starting infertility drugs. Then I had a miscarriage at three months. I have one 15-year-old son.

My sister had her ovaries removed early. Now she has migraines from estrogen replacement therapy.

I've always been underweight.

I have to do something. The doctors want to give me a hysterectomy. I read about homeopathic Sabina. Can it help?

My marriage was awful. It should have lasted only three years, but it lasted 18. I had bad sex with my husband. I later had sex with a male friend about twice a week. When we stopped having sex, the migraines started again. In my current relationship, when we don't see each other (sexually) for three weeks, I get a premenstrual headache (3).

[*There is obviously a hormonal component to her migraines.*]

I get terrible nausea, faintness, and low blood sugar with the headaches (3). The migraines are worse from sunlight (3). I can wake with a headache at 3 a.m. if I didn't wear sunglasses the day before.

My father has always had bad migraines and diabetes. My brother has tension headaches.

I'm very strong-willed (3). I'm an Aries, and I don't let people walk over me (3). I'm hard to be around. I have a hot temper (2). I expect my son to do what I tell him or I yell at him. People say I have high expectations of others and get angry when they don't come through (3). I don't like other people's things to be out of place.

"Patience" is not in my vocabulary (3).

[*She has kind of a dry sarcastic wit, as did the woman in Case Number 2. She is quite entertaining.*]

I've been accused of seeing everything black and white.

[*Doesn't this make you think of the Kali family of remedies?*]

There aren't many people with my personality type. I do have very strong opinions (3). I'll argue with anyone at the drop of a hat if they don't agree with me (3). People say, "You think you're always right."

My childhood was sheltered and repressed. I was in the Peace Corps from 1971 through 1974. I had bad headaches there. I'd never been camping before. I was looking for adventure. I went with my husband.

I recently started my own business. I'm a manufacturer's representative for furniture companies. I approached them and offered to do it.

I'm 45 and have never succeeded at anything (3). I'm afraid of success. I feel almost like I'm an imposter, like I present myself as successful and upbeat but I have a list of failures behind me. I was a teacher for a year, but didn't like it.

I'm a liberated woman. I was furious all the time in Fiji.

[*She felt the culture in Fiji was very sexist.*]

I stayed in real estate for 1½ years, and then left. I started feeling afraid of success. Then I got into the jewelry business.

I'm 45 and the money is running out. I have to succeed.

My son isn't as fond of me as of his father. I begged to get pregnant with him. My ex-husband didn't want kids.

I'm cold (2), except I "bake" at night (3). I can't wear flannel nightgowns. I have to throw the covers off (3). I had hot flashes for three years. If I'm overheated at night I'll wake with a headache.

I like chocolate chip mint ice cream (3), peaches and strawberries (3), and eggnog (3).

I get heartburn from spicy food (2). Coffee goes right through me.

I've started being itchy all over (2) the past year. There's no rash. I've had little red dots on my body since I was exposed to body powder 20 years ago.

My ears have been very sensitive to pierced earrings during the past year.

I was the second of five children.

I still think of myself as "the big girl." I was a foot taller than everyone when I was growing up. They used to call me bossy.

I have two small fibroids. They're heart-shaped.

Observation: She has a pale face.

Assessment: Menorrhagia. I used the following rubrics and symptoms:

- FEMALE, Metrorrhagia, painless.
- MIND, Undertakes many things, perseveres in nothing.
- Headaches, worse from light, menses.
- Menses clotted.
- Pale face.
- Sees things black and white.
- Irritability.

Plan: 1. Kali ferrocyanatum 200c, single dose.
   2. Return after two periods.

Follow-Up on Case Number 3

February 7, 1994

In September and October my periods came every 24 days. Now they're every 28 days. It's leveled out well.

Every month I see more improvement.

I don't have huge clots anymore. They used to be like chicken livers. Now they're the size of quarters, and not that many.

I'm not flooding like before.

Now I'm getting cramps for the first time in years. Just the first day.

I drank one cup of coffee.

[*I asked about recurrent dreams.*]

I've had a dream since I was three or four years old. It's about things being very large and heavy. The burden of the world is upon me. There is so much expected of me. I have to move a big heap of sand. Everything is very large. I have to pick up these big books. I hadn't had this dream for years. Then, after taking the remedy, I had it once again. Just once.

[*This dream vividly depicts the way in which Ferrum struggles. Everything is an effort. Everything is a struggle—her relationship with her ex-husband, with her son, with her family, and so on. The image of moving heaps of sand is very important. It expresses the sense of burden or struggle in her life.*

The same idea comes through in her choice of a business. She sells designer furniture. Furniture stores buy only a few pieces at a time, because they are specialty items. Each time I talk with her she conveys the feeling that her business is barely making it and that she is not choosing the easy route.

I asked if this was a theme in her life.]

Things in my life are weighing heavily on me. Life is a big struggle, a heavy burden.

[*Ananda Zaren says of Kali ferrocyanatum: "The weight of the world is on her shoulders."* (Editors' Note: See discussion later in this presentation.)]

I'm very independent (3). I'm alone out here. I'm proud that I can start a business alone, but it's harder. It would be easier if I were with a man, but I'd lose my independence. And I'm not willing to sacrifice my independence (3).

My childhood was severe, repressed. I was pushed into a mold of being a good girl. They were trying to make me quiet and docile—to change my personality. I feel I've spent my whole adult life—the last 5½ years—breaking away from what others wanted of me.

My father's philosophy of life was that we were all going to behave and follow all the rules and regulations. We had to be good all the time. We were not allowed to say a cross word to each other. That was hard, given my temperament. My parents were very controlled. They never said a harsh word to each other.

Assessment: The remedy is correct.

Plan: 1. Wait.
        2. Return after two more periods.

April 4, 1994

I'm still doing really well.

My periods are good.

I broke up with my boyfriend because he didn't communicate.

I'm getting a few more headaches since I haven't been sexually active.

My business is slowly picking up. I'm not worrying about it anymore like I used to.
    My friends tell me I'm surprisingly calm about starting a new business.

Assessment: Continues to do well.

Plan: 1. Wait.
        2. Return in four months.

Kali Ferrocyanatum: What I Have Learned

When I made the prescription for Case Number 1, the only previous exposure I had to Kali ferrocyanatum was hearing Roger Morrison mention it as a remedy for painless menorrhagia. I knew nothing at all about the mental and emotional picture of the remedy. It made sense to me that the woman in the first case would likely have some combination of symptoms of Kali and Ferrum metallicum. In retrospect, I think that I happened upon this remedy for this patient by luck. I later heard Roger present a Kali ferrocyanatum case, at the last Maui seminar (1993), of a woman with anemia from profuse, clotted menorrhagia.

Other names for the remedy are Kali ferrocyanoretum, Kali ferrocyanicum, and Kali ferrocyanate. The literature (Clarke) states clearly that Kali predominates in Kali ferrocyanatum. In the cases that I presented, however, it is the Ferrum rather than the Kali element that I believe is predominant. As we see more cases of this remedy I will be interested in getting feedback from other homeopaths.

In the following paragraphs I summarize what I have learned from various sources about this remedy and its composition.

Information from a ReferenceWorks Search

Clarke:

> Yellow prussiate of potash; potassic ferrocyanide.
>
> The ferrocyanide of potash is prepared "by fusing animal substances such as the cuttings of horns, hoofs, and skins with carbonate of potash in an iron pot" adding water to the crude product.
>
> The Kali element seems the predominating power in this salt.

Hering:

> Sad; inclination to weep.
>
> Menses too frequent and too profuse, or late.
>
> Menorrhagia, three or four ounces a day, painless.
>
> Passive, painless flowing of blood of natural color, rather thin, and causing much debility.
>
> Pain in small of back, accompanying leucorrhea.

Complete Repertory (Van Zandvoort)

MIND (These are the only mental symptoms in 20,000 rubrics.)
- Ailments from, autumn, mental or emotional symptoms.
- Ailments from, grief, cry, cannot.
- Anger, irascibility, menses, before.
- Anxiety, stomach, in.
- Dreams, amorous.
- Fear, death, of.

- Grief, silent.
- Irritability, easily.
- Irritability, family, to her.
- Irritability, menses, before.
- Sadness.
- Sadness, anger, alternating with.
- Touched, aversion to being.
- Weeping, tearful mood.

FEMALE

- Induration, uterus, cervix, os, and.
- Leucorrhea.
- Leucorrhea, daytime, aggravates, menses, after.
- Leucorrhea, bland.
- Leucorrhea, copious.
- Leucorrhea, cream, like.
- Leucorrhea, menses, after, daytime, usually in.
- Leucorrhea, purulent.
- Leucorrhea, yellow.
- Menses, copious.
- Menses, frequent, too early, too soon.
- Menses, late, too.
- Menses, maroon colored.
- Menses, painful, dysmenorrhea.
- Menses, painful, dysmenorrhea, flow ameliorated.
- Metrorrhagia.
- Metrorrhagia, anemia in.
- Metrorrhagia, painless.
- Metrorrhagia, passive.
- Pain, bearing down.
- Pain, bearing down, uterus, and region of.
- Pregnancy.
- Sexual desire, increased.
- Tumors, ovaries, right.
- Tumors, ovaries, cysts.

Descriptions of Cyanide

From *The Kirk-Othmer Encyclopedia of Chemical Technology*

> Hydrogen cyanide is a colorless, poisonous, low viscosity liquid with an odor characteristic of bitter almonds (which reminds us of laetrile). It is an acute rather than a cumulative poison. It is theorized that hydrocyanide played a key role in animal and plant life on earth via amino acids. It is used extensively in technology. The original source was beet sugar, but now it is synthesized from ammonia and hydrocarbons.

From *The Pharmacologic Basis of Therapeutics* by Goodman and Gilman

> Hydrocyanide is used to fumigate ships and buildings and to sterilize soil. It has a very high affinity for iron in the ferric state. When absorbed, it acts readily with trivalent iron in the mitochondria. Following a transient respiratory stimulation due to decreased oxygenation, cellular respiration is inhibited and cytotoxic hypoxia results. Once the utilization of oxygen is blocked, venous blood is oxygenated and is almost as bright red as arterial blood.

Information from Ananda Zaren

Around the time of the Maui seminar I attended a seminar with Ananda Zaren. She has successfully prescribed Kali ferrocyanatum a number of times. She offered the following information about the remedy based on her clinical experience. She did not give any source references that I can pass on to you.

- Flushes of heat extending upwards.
- Red face with perspiration.
- Menses more frequent around menopause.
- Anemia from metrorrhagia.
- Very heavy menses.
- Bearing down sensation with menses, and gastric sinking.
- Very self-critical, as if she's committed a crime. Judges herself unmercifully.
- Irritability and anxiety.
- Wants to be correct in the eyes of others.
- Hard-working, domineering, industrious (almost workaholic), righteous.

- Preoccupation with what she should do.
- Rarely asks what she wants out of life.
- Her natural wishes were forbidden when she was young. She focused her attention on the correct thing to do rather than on her own desires.
- Deeply resents others who seem to be breaking rules (Kali).
- Chronic resentment and irritability.
- When she goes to bed, she dwells on all the things that have irritated her.
- When angry, she tightens her jaw, purses her lip, and holds her critical words in check.
- Sees anger as a bad emotion.
- Holds grudges and finds it hard to forgive.
- Controlled and controlling.
- Her heart is breaking inside and her uterus is bleeding outside.
- The weight of the world is on her shoulders.

Information from Rajan Sankaran

Spending this January studying with Rajan Sankaran and his colleagues in Bombay helped me to understand the Ferrum aspect of this remedy much more fully. Here are a few ideas from Rajan's new book, *The Substance of Homeopathy*.

Themes of Ferrum metallicum:

- Being compelled to do things against his wishes.
- Fighting against it.
- Guilt of not obeying parents.

Main symptoms of Ferrum:

- Insulting behavior.
- Ailments from anger, vexation, excitement, and scorn.
- Anger from contradiction.
- Anxiety of conscience as if guilty of a crime.
- Company, aversion to, of intimate friends.
- Conscientious.
- Delusions, war, being at.
- Dictatorial.
- Irresolution.
- Occupation ameliorates.

- Quarrelsome.
- Weeping.

Dreams of Ferrum:

- Battles.
- Dead friends and relatives.
- Falling into water.
- Fights.
- War.

Summary Comments

Each of the three cases I have presented share a similar history of emotional repression, of being forced to become a "good girl." The parents were dominating, especially the father. Each woman was in a situation where she could not be herself. She had to fit into a certain mold. "I was pushed into a mold of being a good girl," said the woman in Case Number 3. Yet they also share a very strong need for independence—a need to take action. They did not assert this independence until later in their lives and their road might have been a hard one to travel, but now they are no longer willing to be "molded." These are elements of the Ferrum struggle against repression.

Kali has to do with the family. The Bombay homeopaths we studied with say that Kali involves fighting with the family. Phatak says of Kali carbonicum, "...quarrels with his bread and butter." So, if Kali represents family-quarrel and if Ferrum represents repression-struggle, then perhaps Kali ferrocyanatum translates as struggles against repression from the family.

I'd like to hear from anybody else who has prescribed this remedy to find out your impressions, your experiences with any related remedies, and so on. And I am happy to answer any other questions that you might have.

Roger Morrison: I have had two or three cases of Kali ferrocyanatum. From those cases, I can confirm everything you have said concerning the main elements of this remedy.

Jennifer Jacobs: Well, I want to thank you, Judyth, for giving us such interesting cases and helping to expand our understanding of this lesser-

known remedy. I do have a couple of questions. First of all, I think it is a fairly common experience in our culture for women to be raised in a repressive way, having to be a "good girl" and fit into a mold. There are probably other remedies that have this in their background. Can you differentiate between this remedy and Natrum muriaticum, for example, or some of the other remedies that also have this kind of history? Is there a peculiar aspect of Kali ferrocyanatum in its reaction to that particular type of socialization that could differentiate it from other remedies?

Reichenberg-Ullman: I have to say honestly that what led me to the remedy in all these cases was the painless metrorrhagia. I don't know that I would have selected the remedy just from the mental state. So, I am not sure that I can really answer your question well. However, what I am learning about Ferrum is the idea of a battle. Ferrum dreams of battles. If you go through the mind section of the repertory, looking for Ferrum, you find many rubrics having to do with war, battles, and fighting in the dreams, delusions, and so on. There is a very quarrelsome nature to the Ferrum element that is, I think, a little different from the other remedies that you mentioned. What I can't really describe is the exact difference in the quarrelsome nature of the Kali element, as they talk about it in India, and the Ferrum element.

Jennifer Jacobs: It always happens to me at these conferences that I am reminded of a case I have been working on, where the remedy being presented seems to fit my case. I have one woman patient with heavy bleeding. I have given her Ferrum, and it didn't really help. She came in recently with a swelling around her eyes, especially under the eyebrows, and I gave her Kali carbonicum. But now I am wondering. Have you or anybody else here seen this kind of swelling around the eyes in Kali ferrocyanatum?

Roger Morrison: Yes, I have seen this.

Nancy Herrick: Yes, I think you can see this symptom in all the Kali patients.

Ahmed Currim: Could you tell me if you have used this remedy for men? Certainly, this aspect of struggle is often found in men.

Reichenberg-Ullman: I haven't seen it in men. I have seen these three cases only.

Jane Bernstein: Have you seen the indications that you have described in a patient with a previous hysterectomy and a history of painful periods. Would these symptoms lead you away from thinking of this remedy?

Reichenberg-Ullman: To my way of thinking, if it is really a deep prescription for that person I would expect that she would have needed the remedy for a long time. She probably would have had a long history of painless or close to painless periods. If she had some pain, I wouldn't refrain from giving it. But if she had a lot of pain, I would question the prescription. I just don't think this remedy would be likely to manifest in that way very often.

Karl Robinson: Would you prescribe it if there was no metrorrhagia and it wasn't painless? [audience laughter]

Reichenberg-Ullman: Sure, if it fit the case.

Karl Robinson: Really? [audience laughter] Even if the patient came in with other complaints?

Reichenberg-Ullman: I would.

Karl Robinson: Okay. [Audience laughter.] It's just that this is one of those remedies where all that has been handed down to us is this one primary symptom of painless metrorrhagia. That is what the remedy is known for.

Reichenberg-Ullman: Yes, definitely. But, as you know, Karl, from having also studied in India, there are plenty of cases where the physical pathology of the person is not in the repertory, yet the remedy, prescribed solely on the mental and general symptoms, still works for the case. Maybe I wouldn't actually be able to perceive the remedy on the mental and general symptoms alone, because of a limited amount of understanding at this point. Or maybe this is really a very small remedy that is indicated only in these cases of metrorrhagia, as we now believe it to be. It may be our limited knowledge. Has anyone here given this remedy for other situations?

Roger Morrison: Yes, I used it in a case of asthma with very good results. The prescription was based on many of the same ideas that Judyth is talking about, especially the aggressiveness of the Ferrum element. The central pathology was asthma. This woman did have heavy menstrual periods, but it wasn't her main problem. The heavy periods were an ancillary symptom.

Reichenberg-Ullman: Do you remember, Roger, whether they were painless periods?

Roger Morrison: They were not really painful, neither very painful nor outstandingly painless. I want to make one other comment. There was a good article on Ferrum in Homeopathic Links *a couple of years ago. The term "iron will" was used to describe the remedy, and it was interesting that one of your patients said she had a "cast iron" stomach.*

David Riley, MD

THREE CASES OF INFERTILITY OF INFERTILITY AND PELVIC INFLAMMATORY DISEASE (PID)

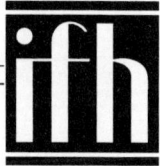

David Riley is board-certified in Internal Medicine and a graduate of the Hahnemann College of Homeopathy. He lives in Santa Fe, New Mexico, where he practices homeopathy and is conducting an ongoing series of classical homeopathic drug provings.

An Introduction to Thiosinaminum
(Derived from Oil of Mustard)

This remedy has been effective in curing adhesions, cicatrices, lupus, enlarged lymphatic glands, stricture of rectum, tinnitus aurium, and tumors of the uterus appendages. We need provings of this medicine; it has great possibilities of cure in serious conditions of disease.

—Grimmer

I had the good fortune of being introduced to this remedy in 1987. It was mentioned in passing by another homeopath. About one year later I used it successfully for one patient, and over the years I have used it with some success for five other patients with a variety of conditions. As I was preparing this presentation I was surprised to discover that I had used this remedy 12 times.

The most striking cases in terms of consistent results were three cases of infertility secondary to pelvic inflammatory disease. The patients in these cases had several symptoms in common: the appearance of scarring (particularly pelvic scarring), in conjunction with depression, alternating moods, and aversion to consolation. They also had confirmatory symptoms of seasonal allergies and increased urination at night.

The title of this presentation refers to the three successful Thiosinaminum prescriptions in the first two cases. (Case Number 2 actually contains two successful Thiosinaminum prescriptions, resulting in pregnancies 1½ years apart.) In Case Number 3, the patient has not yet become pregnant, but she has made significant progress on the mental and emotional levels after receiving Thiosinaminum.

I will also briefly present two more cases in which I have used Thiosinaminum with considerable benefit. Each case, although more or less a keynote prescription, is quite interesting and demonstrates the wider range of therapeutic uses of the remedy. The positive result in each case was confirmed by a follow-up diagnostic exam.

In the past two years I have been consciously trying to explore and develop some of the edges of this remedy on several levels. I have attempted to pay more attention to characteristics other than physical scarring that may be associated with the remedy, including the possibility of depression involving emotional "scarring." But I must admit that this remedy still enters into my differential diagnosis primarily on the basis of physical pathology.

I hope that our discussion today will stimulate others to use this remedy so that we can refine our collective understanding of it. One of the most difficult aspects of using the remedy is learning how to pronounce and spell it! It wasn't until I prepared this talk that I was able to consistently do this correctly.

[Editors' Note: Dr. Riley's spontaneous comments, made while presenting his cases, are bracketed and italicized.]

Case Number 1

Female
Age 34

Initial Visit: April 1988

Chief Complaints:
- Rash on her arms and chest (1).
- Infertility, presumably secondary to pelvic inflammatory disease (PID) (2).

[*PID, or pelvic inflammatory disease, is a kind of sexually transmitted disease in which women develop an inflammation of the fallopian tubes. The fallopian tubes contain a series of small hairs or cilia that beat downstream from the ovaries toward the uterus. After the egg leaves the ovary it moves into the fallopian tubes, and the cilia move the egg down the fallopian tube. Conception usually occurs in the tube, and then the cilia move the fertilized egg into the uterus, where implantation occurs.*

PID can be the result of any number of infectious etiologies. When a woman contracts gonorrhea, for example, the cilia in the fallopian tube may be destroyed and they frequently do not regenerate. The process of destruction can result in scarring and a narrowing or complete obstruction of the fallopian tube. This tube does not have a large caliber to begin with. Basically, if you were to see a fallopian tube you would not be able to find the opening in it. It is more of a potential space that is there when the egg passes through on the way to the uterus. The patency of the tube can be checked by doing what is called a hysterosalpingogram, involving the injection of dye.]

She is a strikingly eccentric (3) woman who had been a filmmaker in Los Angeles before moving to New Mexico. She couldn't stand the fast-paced and superficial lifestyle of the film industry and Los Angeles. She is a loner (3), seemingly by choice, but she claims it is because there is no one she can relate to. She had been reasonably successful, producing two films and receiving support from several well-known actors before she moved.

She is moody (3) and easily hurt and offended, although she usually keeps this well hidden. When she is moody she wants to eat (2).

She is depressed in general (3) over her inability to be successful in the world and with her inability to manifest what she wants out of life—a functional relationship, a family, and a successful career.

She has raised bloodhounds for many years. It could be said that her closest relationships are with her dogs.

She lives in what appears to be a poverty-stricken state, surrounded by yelping bloodhounds, in a trailer in the middle of nowhere on the wind-swept high desert plains south of Santa Fe.

She supports herself by working odd jobs here and there and by slowly selling her assets, some of which are valuable, to local art dealers in northern New Mexico.

Two months ago she met a man who spoke no English (Japanese), married him two months later, and now wants to have children.

She had two previous episodes of PID, had an abnormal hysterosalpingogram, and had been told that she would never be able to get pregnant. Because she has no health insurance and not much money, in vitro fertilization is out of the question.

"I can't relate to the world. I never have been very good at that" (3). I sometimes think I am great, and other times I think I am worthless. Sometimes I just want to be left alone, but I hate that too" (3).

Observation: She is closed and shy, watching me carefully (3).

Didn't get along with her parents when she was growing up; refuses to visit them now (2).

Warm-blooded (1).

Suffers from allergies in the spring (constant coryza) (3).

Desires spicy (3), salty (3), and sour foods (1). Increased appetite (3).

Thirsty; prefers cold drinks (1).

Experiences cramping, pain, and heavy bleeding (3) with her menses. The pain varies from menses to menses (2).

Increased urination at night (2).

She has a long history of herpes, but hasn't had any outbreaks in nine months (1).

A barely visible, minimally red rash appears on her shoulders and chest. It does not itch, and does not really bother her at all (1).

Her sleep is fine, except when she is wakened by her dogs. She dreams of her dogs (1).

Analysis of Case Number 1

The prominent elements are on two levels: infertility secondary to PID on the physical level and an inability to cope with the world on the mental level. This inability is manifested by moodiness, a history of depression, and an eccentric lifestyle. Her moodiness is further characterized by its changeability and her tendency to overreact.

I considered Sulphur, because of her general state, and Lac caninum, because of the specific symptoms. However, I decided to try a one-month course of Thiosinaminum, a prescription based largely on the physical pathology of pelvic scarring (PID).

Plan: Thiosinaminum 12c, daily.

Follow-Up on Case Number 1

June 1988

The rash disappeared the first week after taking the remedy.

She is now three weeks pregnant.

She is not moody or depressed. Excited about being pregnant.

She is learning Japanese so she can talk with her husband.

Plan: Wait.

May 1989

She has a healthy baby boy.

No recurrence of symptoms.

Plan: Wait.

Long-Term Follow-Up

She has subsequently gone on to have two other children with her husband. She is still married and living happily as far as I know. My last contact with her was in 1991, before she moved out of the area.

Additional Comments on Case Number 1

This was my first Thiosinaminum case. I must say I didn't have much confidence in my prescription when I gave it. It seemed like a reasonable stab in the dark. However, even after she became pregnant, which I thought was wonderful, I still wondered if it was due to the remedy. Subsequently, I have had other cases with follow-up diagnostic evaluations showing changes in physical pathology and even the disappearance of physical pathology. So, I am no longer in doubt as to the potential efficacy of this remedy.

Audience: Why did you use a low potency, and for how long was the 12c taken?

Riley: The remedy was taken daily for about six weeks. As for the use of low potency, it is my belief, one I am challenging a bit these days, that a "dense" and clearly recognizable physical pathology is like a crystallization of disturbances that exist on other levels. In these situations, the central focus seems to lie somewhere other than on the emotional level, and it has been my practice to give low potency remedies on a repeated basis. I don't always do it that way now, but that was the rationale behind the way I prescribed then.

Case Number 2

Female
Age 40

Initial Visit: January 1992

Chief Complaints:
- Infertility, secondary to PID (3).
- Depression (2).

She is a psychotherapist.

She had used a Dalkon shield, which resulted in PID. Her left fallopian tube was removed in 1980. A hysterosalpingogram showed a blocked fallopian tube on the right side. She had a Gardnerella infection in 1987 (itching and a general sense of discomfort in the pelvis accompanied by a white discharge). It was successfully treated with antibiotics (1).

[*With one fallopian tube removed and the other blocked, the chance of pregnancy by normal means is probably less than 1 percent. The method usually used is in vitro fertilization, in which eggs are harvested, sperm is collected, fertilization is initiated in a test tube, and the fertilized egg is then reimplanted into the uterus. The hope is that the fertilized egg will implant and develop.*]

She has a long history of depression dating back to her childhood (3).

Her mother died when she was four, her father remarried, and her stepmother was physically and verbally abusive. The stepmother was very strict and offered no affection. Frequent beatings. Her parents fought a great deal. She used to withdraw and wish her real mother were there instead of the stepmother. She was depressed, withdrawn, and angry at the world for taking away her mother (3). She left home as a rebellious teenager. Her mother's death left a deep emotional scar, and she has worked hard to overcome it.

She was married once before and has been married for six years to her second husband. She is very happy in her relationship now but still likes to have time alone (3).

She currently experiences a seasonal affective disorder (3), which has generally improved since moving to New Mexico.

(She is quiet with a melancholic demeanor and gives the impression of having suffered a great deal of emotional trauma in her life.)

Her menstrual cycle is regular (28 days) with no PMS either now or in the past. History of irregular menses (one to two days early or late).

"I have a hard time trusting people, and I usually am on guard at first to try to prevent others from hurting me" (3).

She is not averse to consolation now but still has the impulse to be alone when upset (3).

Afraid of being hurt (3), attacked/raped (3), being alone—yet often prefers to be alone (3), and the dark (2). Also claustrophobic (2).

Suffers from allergies (runny nose and itchy eyes) in the spring (1).

Has a tendency toward constipation (2).

Long history of severe hemorrhoids (3).

Desires chocolate (3). She is mostly vegetarian and has a big appetite (3).

Thirsty for cold drinks. She frequently has a parched throat in the summer.

Intermittent increased urination (2). Old history of urinary tract infections (1).

Her sleep is generally good except when she is alone; then, she wakes easily.

She dreams of being stuck somewhere and she can't move (3). She also dreams of robbers (2).

She is generally chilly (2), especially her hands and feet.

She is averse to consolation when angry and could get really angry or moody if she did not have interpersonal skills to pull her through (3).

Analysis of Case Number 2

As in Case Number 1, depression and a closed, serious demeanor were prominent threads running through the case. Yet, it was clear to me that the key issue for her was infertility. Given the previous case where there was a history of pelvic scarring I chose to give Thiosinaminum, which ended up working well. (It is interesting to note that she also had positive responses to Ignatia and Natrum muriaticum during the course of her treatment.)

Plan: Thiosinaminum 12c, daily.

Follow-Up on Case Number 2

March 1992

Her old sense of impending depression is gone.

She is pregnant.

No allergies this spring.

Plan: Wait.

May 1992

She had a miscarriage: deep grief, depression, occasional emotional outbursts.

A follow-up hysterosalpingogram showed a patent fallopian tube on the right side.

[*I was quite impressed with the results of the hysterosalpingogram, because this was not supposed to be possible! I discussed it with the gynecologist, who was somewhat interested in what it was I had done. I told her that it was a very obscure remedy with a keynote for pelvic scarring and that I did not have much experience with it.*]

Plan: Ignatia 200c, single dose, for her acute state.

June 1992

She has been much better since taking the remedy.

No hysteria, but she is still depressed.

Plan: Natrum muriaticum 1M, single dose.

[*I had thought of giving Natrum muriaticum at the first visit if Thiosinaminum had not worked for her.*]

June 1993

She is not able to get pregnant (no hysterosalpingogram).

No depression; a big change after taking the Natrum muriaticum. Emotional improvement was immediate and sustained.

No spring allergies.

Plan: Thiosinaminum 12c, daily.

September 1993

She is pregnant.

(She later delivered a baby girl.)

Long-Term Follow-Up

This patient has had no recurrence of the depression and no recurrence of the spring allergies. The disappearance of her allergies was really what caused me to begin paying considerably more attention to the remedy.

Case Number 3

Female
Age 42

Initial Visit: April 1993

She has a long history of infertility (3), abdominal pain (3), and gynecological problems.

She was just told that she might be going into premature menopause and might never be able to get pregnant. She feels a deep sense of grief (3) and loss.

Her marriage may be in jeopardy. She has occasional suicidal thoughts (2) but can't imagine how she could end things. These mood swings may be secondary to the hormonal replacement therapy (Clomid and Perganol) she is undergoing to treat her infertility.

She is normally very goal-oriented, efficient, and upbeat (2).

Multiple adhesions were found in both her ovaries and her left fallopian tube at the time of her surgery for a pelvic abscess in 1992. She was told she had a propensity to form scar tissue and adhesions. Her whole world fell apart at that time (3). Since then, she has suffered from abdominal pain.

[*The doctors said it was one of the worst cases of scarring they had ever seen. She underwent a series of four surgical procedures by laparoscopy over the course of a year, to try to remove as many adhesions as possible. They helped somewhat, but she was still in significant pain when she came to see me.*]

Her menses have not been normal for over a year because of the hormonal therapy. The symptoms she has been experiencing secondary to the hormonal therapy are driving her "crazy." She has hot flashes, mood swings, and other symptoms that seem to be related to the therapy.

Gynecological History:
- Endometriosis (3) since 1980.
- Ovarian cysts (3) first diagnosed in 1982.
- Surgery for pelvic abscess (3) in 1992:
  – Left-sided, walled-off pelvic abscess.
  – Sudden onset.
  – Became hysterical at the time the abscess was discovered (3).

Gets headaches (2).

Acne (3).

Suffers from allergies in the spring and fall; fluent coryza and itchy eyes (3).

She runs a business with her husband. She is the organizational force for the company and is generally a perfectionist (3), but not fastidious.

She feels better from exercise and is athletically inclined (3).

On the whole, she is chilly (2).

She is sensitive to noise (3).

She is averse to consolation (3).

Her sleep is okay.

She dreams of being trapped and not being able to escape (3). Also dreams of surgery (2).

Desires sweets (4), salt (3), and caffeine (3).

She generally is not thirsty. She has to remind herself to drink (2).

She has not been able to conceive for many years. She has been trying to get pregnant for two years.

She feels she is going crazy (3). Feels hysterical (3) and suicidal (2).

Her husband has said that he may leave if she can't get pregnant.

Analysis of Case Number 3

There is significant mental pathology. It all seems to originate from the difficulties in conceiving and can be partly attributed to the hormonal therapy administered to induce pregnancy. The most interesting point in this case is that her depression is relieved from the remedy even though she does not become pregnant.

Plan: Thiosinaminum 200c, plus 12c daily.

Follow-Up on Case Number 3

June 1993

After taking the remedy she noticed a sense of detachment from her grief and sadness. For one week she tried to recreate the depressed mood before finally resigning herself to feeling okay despite the possible "tragedy" of premature menopause.

After the second week she started enjoying an increased sense of well-being, even though the external circumstances of her life have changed little.

She feels that her abdomen is "loosening up." It is as if "the outside of my skin and actual size are the same but there is more of me inside. I can feel myself more and it feels okay."

[*The abdominal pain was significantly better. Initially, she had graded the pain as a "7" or "8" on a scale of 10. At this first follow-up she graded it as a "2" or "3."*]

She feels less constriction and tightness in her pelvis and lower back.

No headaches (2).

Less chilly (3).

She started therapy (again) with her husband. (I spoke with her therapist who said that in the past she was very moody and capable of going into rages. She seems more connected with herself and the world around her now, according to the therapist.)

Plan: Continue Thiosinaminum 12c, daily. (She is still on hormonal therapy.)

October 1993

She stopped taking the Thiosinaminum in mid-September and noted an increase in abdominal pain after two weeks. So she began taking the 12c daily once again. The abdominal pain resolved after restarting the remedy.

She is experiencing a general increase in strength and stamina.

Her marriage is going better; her business is going better.

She is going to begin a new experimental infertility program in Albuquerque next month.

She still feels sad about her inability to conceive. She feels that she is supposed to have children and tries to remain hopeful about pregnancy. Also feels that she has let down her husband but has difficulty talking with him about this.

Plan: Thiosinaminum 200c, single dose.

March 1994

She is stopping the infertility program.

Her abdominal pain is still gone.

She is exercising more.

Her business is going well.

She is less depressed.

Plan: Wait.

Case Number 4

Male
Age 37

Initial Visit: March 1993

Chief Complaints:
- Alcohol abuse (3).
- Rectal stricture (2).

This man came to me two days before he was scheduled to have part of his colon surgically removed.

He had a long history of alcohol abuse, and he had been in a number of treatment programs. He had recently gone on an extensive alcoholic binge, after the woman he was in a relationship with had left him.

He is semi-employed.

He had ended up in a hospital treatment program.

While in recovery, he began to have significant abdominal pain. The psychiatrist referred him for a barium enema and lower GI series. They were not able to perform the procedure because the dye could not pass. There was a stricture. The surgeon told him it would be necessary to remove the affected part of the colon, a length of six to twelve inches. He wasn't terribly excited about that and was looking for an alternative.

Plan: 1. Nux vomica 200c, single dose.
2. Liquid diet: vegetable juices and broth.
3. Appropriate yoga postures.

Follow-Up on Case Number 4

First Follow-Up

He recovered quite nicely.

The pain subsided and he is able to have normal stools.

He is quite happy with the results and is doing well generally.

He has found work again.

June 1993

He is continuing to do well.

He has three to four formed stools per day without straining, which is normal bowel function for him.

Assessment: We agreed that he was doing fine. I felt the Nux vomica was working and that no other remedy was needed at the moment. I explained to him, however, that I still recommended that he have diagnostic flexible sigmoidoscopy at some point in the near future, because the original procedure had never been successfully completed.

Plan: Wait.

November 1993

The sigmoidoscopy, performed in November 1993, revealed a one to two centimeter diameter stricture at the junction of the descending and sigmoid colon. No other abnormalities were noted. The doctors all strongly recommended that he have the stricture surgically removed.

He continues to have three to four formed stools per day.

He is optimistic and happy.

He is not drinking alcohol.

No other complaints.

Plan: Thiosinaminum 12c, daily for two months.

April 1994

A follow-up flexible sigmoidoscopy showed a resolution of the stricture. No abnormality could be found.

> *Barbara Newlon: When you saw the patient three months after the original Nux vomica prescription, was he experiencing any bowel problems or any other problem at the time?*

> *Riley: No. He felt that his life had returned to normal. He had normal bowel function.*

> *Barbara Newlon: During that initial three-month period, had his alcoholism changed?*

> *Riley: Well, he had been in a treatment program. He hadn't had a drink. He had found a job, albeit not a great job. He was working as a parking lot attendant at a local hotel. Later on, his job fortunes improved. The last I heard from him, he was a stockbroker and he was developing a software program.*

> *Barbara Newlon: So, the only thing you were concerned about at the three-month follow-up was the frequent stools, three to four per day?*

> *Riley: At the three-month follow-up, I wasn't concerned at all. He was doing quite well. The stools were well-formed, and he was not complaining about anything else. I do think that most people do not have three to four bowel movements a day, but, once again, he had no complaints about them. He was working, and his diet was good. He was in an optimistic mood. He wasn't drinking at all. I was happy with what was going on with him from a homeopathic point of view.*

> *However, I was interested in getting the flexible sigmoidoscopy done at some point to find out what was going on in the colon. The diagnosis of cancer was entertained initially. And, so, it was in the back of my mind that he might really have colon cancer or something of this nature. I felt I should be following up on this. I have certain liabilities in terms of diagnostics.*

> *Barbara Newlon: Well, I think it is an important point. When we see a curative response on many levels from a remedy, I don't think very many*

people in this room would have thought to do what you did, in ordering the sigmoidoscopy.

Riley: *I would have to say that much of it was the liability issue. He had been seen by several people in the local medical community, people who are my colleagues and even friends in some cases. The surgeon who was going to operate on him is someone I like a great deal. He was very interested in what was going on with the homeopathic treatment. I had maintained correspondence with all his various caregivers. I thought I needed to order the test to have a complete picture of what, in fact, was going on, because the diagnostic procedure that had led to the recommendation for surgery in the first place had never been successfully performed. From a pathological point of view, we didn't know what was happening in his colon. I was expecting the sigmoidoscopy to be normal.*

Case Number 5

Let me briefly describe one more case in which I have recently used Thiosinaminum. From a general homeopathic point of view, I haven't really gotten anywhere with this patient. With Thiosinaminum, I have helped him on a relatively minor acute level. The patient is happy, while I am relatively dissatisfied with the overall case. However, the result after Thiosinaminum is noteworthy.

Male
Age 46

I began seeing him in May 1993. I persisted in prescribing Lycopodium for him without any results at all. He comes back dutifully at regular intervals and tells me he has had no success at all with the remedy. I am still convinced he needs Lycopodium, but that is probably my "delusion," not his (audience laughter)!

About three months ago, he brought up a problem he had not mentioned before. It is a ringing in the ears that has been occurring for the past year, getting worse recently. He had seen an ear, nose, and throat specialist, whose examination revealed a 70 percent hearing loss in the right ear. The diagnosis was otosclerosis.

In March of this year (1994), I prescribed Thiosinaminum 12c, to be taken daily, based solely on the physical pathology. He reported a significant subjective improvement. He said the ringing in his ears was 50 percent improved and his hearing was much better. His specialist re-examined him and found a 30 to 40 percent improvement in the hearing of the right ear.

Thiosinaminum/Mustard: Results of a ReferenceWorks Search

Boedler/Bach

Mustard treats states of depression and gloom.

MIND. While being in the Mustard state, the mind is overshadowed by darkness and gloom, and there may be the sensation of a weight or downward pull that depresses the person as a whole. The mind actually appears to receive less light, and the person cheers up in the warm, bright rays of the sun. People who crave light and sunshine are often in need of this remedy. Bach describes this state as a sensation of a dark cloud which descends, sometimes for inexplicable reasons.

The depressive character of this state makes the person turn inward, as if locked within, and the connection to the outside world is weakened. It takes effort to perk up and lift oneself out of this state; one may appear as absent-minded, introverted, or disinterested in present circumstances. Cheerfulness or lightness of being are not easily achieved under these circumstances. Life does not appeal; tasks and interaction with people seem to give no incentive or joy. In depressive disorders, this remedy helps to bring about cure. In retardation, Mustard can help alleviate withdrawal and joylessness.

EMOTIONS. Depression and gloom may bring the emotions of sadness, regret, boredom, self-pity, weepiness, and a sense of meaninglessness. Or one may be morose and ill-tempered, seeking to retreat from involvement with others, while succumbing to gloom. In severe cases, there may also be despair and a sense of desolation, of loneliness. One may feel as an island, life holds no incentive, while other people seem busy and cheered. The purpose of existence is veiled in the Mustard state. Life seems to stagnate, and aspirations lie dormant.

In lighter cases, depression does not seem so overbearing, but rather like a passing mood that reasserts from time to time. Some experiences, such as failure, sadness, or regret may bring on the Mustard state. At other times, the dark cloud descends unannounced, without apparent reason, to stifle the joy of the day. Here too, a lack of meaningful occupation, based on dormant potentials and unrecognized soul purpose in work and human relations, may lie at the root of the problem.

PHYSICAL TENDENCIES. Depression may lead to lowered vitality, lethargy, chronic fatigue, and appetite disturbances, resulting in either weight loss or gain and constipation. There may also be sleeping disturbances, disinterest in physical recreation, and general decline in healthful interests and habits. A head injury can be a mechanical reason for the appearance of the Mustard state. Nerve damage or misalignment of skull plates along fissures may dampen consciousness which may not be able to receive as much brightness and light as before the accident.

DOCTRINE OF SIGNATURES. The yellow Mustard plant spreads across the land profusely, reminding of the cheer-bringing rays of the sun. The plant usually grows above other grasses and weeds in the field, reminding of its healing quality to uplift and raise the mind above gloom. It also gives the idea of lightness and joy, not only by its color but also by its light dance in the breeze.

[*Mustard grows wild in New Mexico, and it is quite a beautiful plant. It usually comes up late in the spring after other plants have already appeared. The countryside in New Mexico is barren much of the time. In the spring, a veneer of grasses and other plants starts to grow. At some point in the spring the mustard plant comes up through all of this, creating a wonderful yellow hue in the fields. It is an aggressive plant.*]

Mustard seeds have the tendency to lie dormant in the ground for many years. They suddenly spring up when the conditions for growth are right. This is usually after the ground has been freshly ploughed. Similarly, human potentials and talents may lie buried at the bottom of the inner self, preventing the soul's sparks of joy and meaningfulness from germinating. Ploughing the inner self in the process of self-discovery, usually brought forth through the experience of the self in and through the world and its people, will help to air one's inner treasures. In biblical terms, the Mustard seed is used as a symbol of the inner kingdom of grace which grows to bring joy and fulfillment to the soul.

Anschutz

Rhodallin, allyl sulphocarbamide. Prepared for homeopathic use by trituration with milk sugar.

The following was contributed by Alfred M. Moore, MD, Brighton, Colorado, 1910:

The treatment of tinnitus aurium has long been so unsatisfactory that the rule to make no promises has been fixed among men who have had any experience with that distressing condition. I have made many attempts to give relief to those applying with the various noises in their ears, but not until I began the use of Thiosinaminum was I able to get any result whatever in the cases of long standing. My attention was directed to this drug by an article published in *Practical Medicine*, page 304, issue of 1906, since which time I have been gratified with the results in the treatment of chronic catarrh of the middle ear with or without the tinnitus. However, the greatest result is in cases with the noises which are so annoying; that is, the patient expresses such satisfaction from the relief and also the improvement in hearing.

The article referred to is credited to Dr. McCullogh and his findings are stated as follows: (1) That it exerts a marked beneficial action on ear diseases accompanied by the formation of new connective tissue; (2) that this beneficial action is due to an increased pliability of this tissue; (3) that its administration should always be accompanied by mechanical measures; (4) that better and more prompt results may be obtained in recent cases; (5) that it exerts a beneficial action on vertigo; (6) that better results may be obtained with it in the relief of tinnitus aurium than with any drug used heretofore.

I have verified the above, and in some cases, without the mechanical means for vibrating the membrane tympani, rapid relief has followed its administration. I looked up the literature on this drug, but found practically nothing. Squibb gives its dosage as ½ to 1½ grains three times daily by the mouth. However, I have found that even ½ grain doses produce undesirable symptoms in some individuals, such as nausea, vomiting, pains in the head, and general muscular twitching; but the general statement is that the head is cleared of the fullness and tinnitus, the mucous membrane of the upper respiratory tract being affected beneficially by lessening the secretions, producing a dryness, etc. And I believe that by triturating this remedy to remove from it the crude effects and giving it in the divided dosage, which would doubtless increase the curative effects, we will have found a remedy which will benefit a larger percentage of cases of middle ear diseases, with or without tinnitus, than any heretofore used. May 20th, 1910.

Blackwood

THERAPEUTICS. This remedy has been employed both locally and internally in cases of lupus, chronic enlarged glands, strictures, and for dissolving scar tissue. It has relieved stricture of the rectum, when two grains were given twice a day. Also tinnitus aurium, where the ossicles were bound down by fibrous bands.

Boericke

(A chemical derived from oil of mustard-seed.)

A resolvent, externally and internally, for DISSOLVING SCAR TISSUE, tumors, enlarged glands; lupus, strictures, adhesions. Ectropion, opacities of cornea, cataract, ankylosis, fibroids, scleroderma. Noises in ear. Suggested by Dr. A.S. Hard for retarding old age. A remedy for tabes dorsalis, improving the lightning pains. Gastric, vesicle and rectal crises. Stricture of rectum, 2 grains twice daily.

Arteriosclerotic VERTIGO. TINNITUS. Catarrhal deafness with cicatricial thickening. Subacute suppurative otitis media, formation of fibrous bands impeding free movement of the ossicles. Thickened drum. Deafness due to some fibrous change in the nerve.

Clarke

INTRODUCTION: Allyl sulphocarbamide. (Derived from oil of mustard-seed.) Trituration of the crystals. Solution in alcohol.

CLINICAL:

- Adhesions.
- Cicatrices.
- Lupus.
- Lymphatic glands, enlarged.
- Rectum, stricture of.
- Strictures.
- Tinnitus aurium.
- Tumors.

CHARACTERISTICS: Thiosinaminum belongs to the same chemical group as urea. The colorless bitter crystals are soluble in water, alcohol, and ether.

Thiosinaminum has been used externally and internally in cases of lupus, chronic glandular tumors, and for dissolving scar tissue. Dose in old-school practice is 4 to 8 grains once a day given hypodermically in a 15 percent solution.

C. H. Pennoyer (quoted Pac. C. J. of H. viii. 199) relates this case: Mrs. C., 69, had been several years ill with gastric distress, sciatica, pains in hips down to knees, worse by motion. Indigestion, flatulence of stomach and bowels, worse after eating. Pain in back. Inability to walk, much perspiration, depression of spirits, and subnormal temperature.

Her father had died at 69 of stomach trouble, mother at 58 of stricture of the bowel. Examination showed stricture of rectum two inches above anus, there being a tense fibrous band forming a ring opening, which would not admit the index finger. Bougies and mechanical measures failed to relieve. Weakness was so great, patient would faint at stool. Under general treatment nutrition improved, but the local condition was unchanged.

A year later the stricture was slightly increased.

Thiosinaminum was now given, gr. ii. twice daily.

The following year the patient was found much improved. Examination showed that the cicatricial band had gone, the speculum could be introduced, and the mucous membrane was normal in appearance, though not as distensible as a normal rectum should be.

W. Spencer (H. M., xxxiv. 55) has applied this property of resolving cicatricial tissues in cases of tinnitus aurium "where the ossicles are bound down, and the function of the tympanic cavity so much impaired by fibrous bands or adhesions." In such cases he has had encouraging success.

Enlarged lymphatic glands have been reduced in the same way. A few symptoms observed on patients under treatment I have arranged in the schema with some cured symptoms.

Ears—Tinnitus caused by fibrous bands.

Stomach—Appetite increased.

Rectum—Stricture of rectum resolved.

Urinary Organs—Urine increased in quantity, no albumen or formed elements.

Female Genitalia—Tumors of uterine appendages.

Respiration—Accelerated respiration.

Generalities—Sensation of heat and burning in affected parts. Bodily weight increased. Glandular swellings reduced.

Skin—Distinct local reaction in lupus cases after hours. Urticaria. Lupus. Scar tissues.

Thiosinaminum as Represented in the Repertory

I also used the computer to search for all incidences of Thiosinaminum in the Complete Repertory (by Roger van Zandvoort, in MacRepertory). The remedy appears only 40 times in the entire repertory (Figure 1). Actually, I was surprised to find even that many, so perhaps that is the good news! The bad news would then be that Thiosinaminum does not appear in bold type under any rubric.

It is interesting, as well, to see which remedies are most similar to Thiosinaminum, in terms of the rubrics where it appears (Figure 1). It makes perfect sense, when you think about the physical pathology covered by Thiosinaminum, that the closest remedy would be Silica.

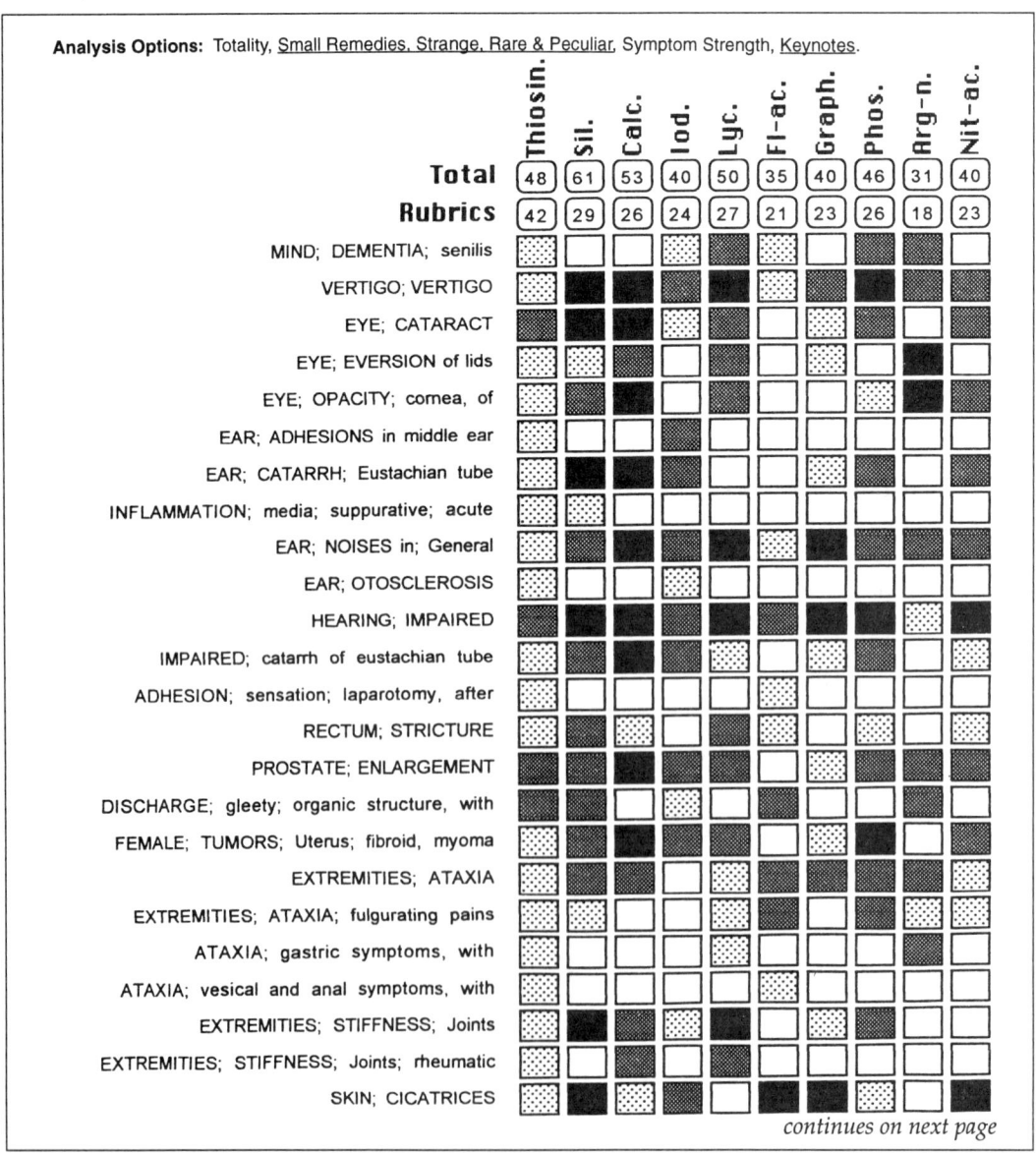

Figure 1
Results of a Repertory Search for Thiosinaminum

Figure 1, *cont'd*

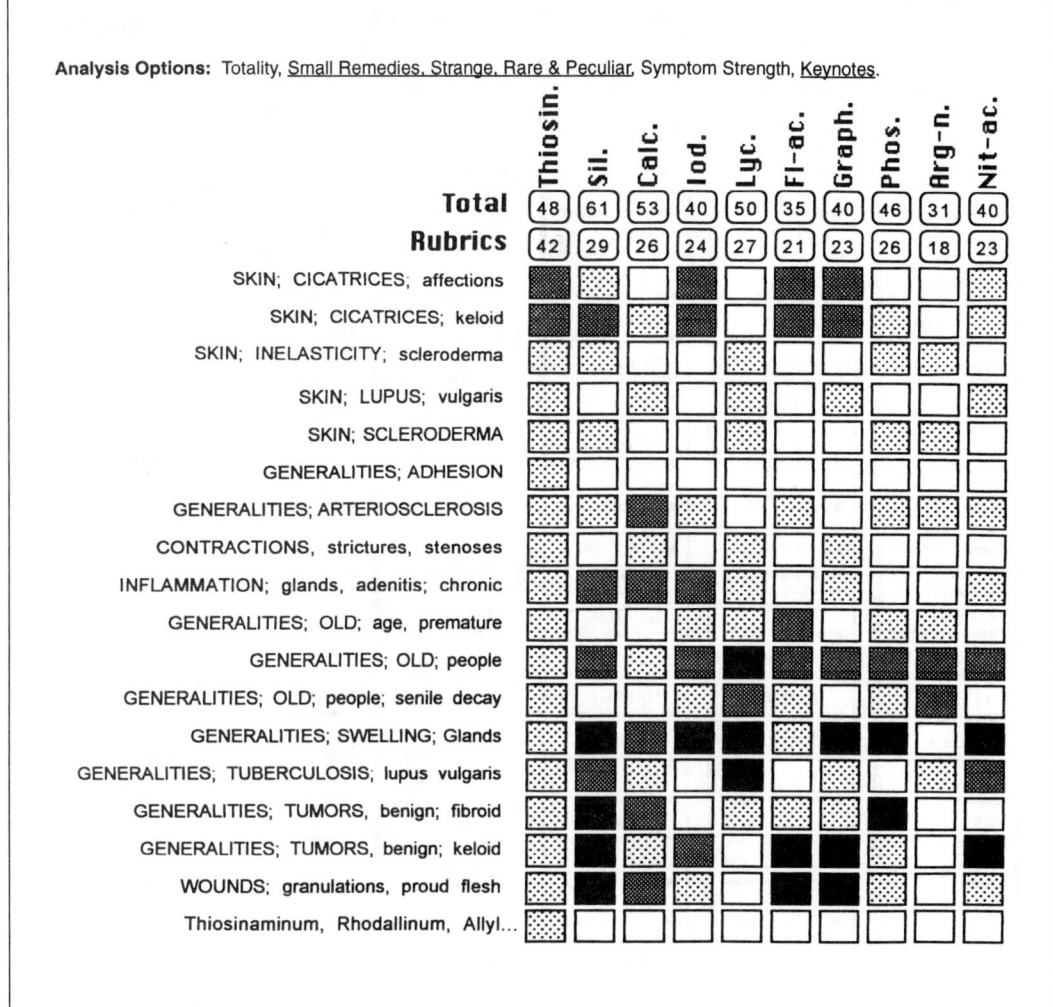

I also used the MacRepertory program to analyze the results of the Thiosinaminum search in terms of the separate categories, Totality; Small Remedies; Strange, Rare, and Peculiar; Symptom Strength; Keynotes; and Number of Rubrics (Figure 2). In several categories, other remedies figure as or more prominently than Thiosinaminum. There seem to be as yet no keynotes that are unique to this remedy.

Totality	Small Remedies	Strange, Rare &	Symptom Strength	Keynotes	Number of Rubrics
84 Sil.	84 Thiosin.	84 Thiosin.	84 Sil.	84 Sil.	84 Thiosin.
72 Calc.	13 Calc-f.	32 Fl-ac.	71 Calc.	84 Thiosin.	57 Sil.
68 Lyc.	12 Fl-ac.	26 Iod.	67 Thiosin.	79 Arg-n.	53 Lyc.
65 Thiosin.	11 Calc-i.	21 Lyc.	64 Lyc.	72 Lyc.	50 Calc.
62 Phos.	10 Iod.	21 Sil.	62 Sulph.	64 Calc.	50 Phos.
61 Sulph.	10 Thyr.	18 Calc.	61 Phos.	64 Iod.	49 Ars.
54 Graph.	9 Bar-m.	16 Arg-n.	56 Iod.	60 Phos.	49 Sulph.
54 Iod.	9 Hydrc.	14 Graph.	55 Graph.	59 Puls.	47 Iod.
54 Nit-ac.	9 Tub.	13 Iris-t.	55 Nit-ac.	52 Ars.	44 Graph.
53 Ars.	8 Agn.	13 Phos.	50 Caust.	52 Fl-ac.	44 Nit-ac.
50 Con.	8 Ars-i.	12 Ars.	49 Con.	51 Rhus-t.	41 Fl-ac.
47 Caust.	8 Aur-i.	12 Caust.	48 Ars.	46 Nux-v.	38 Caust.
47 Fl-ac.	8 Ferr-pic.	12 Nux-v.	48 Fl-ac.	45 Graph.	38 Lach.
46 Bell.	8 Hydr.	12 Sulph.	47 Merc.	43 Alum.	38 Merc.
46 Merc.	8 Kres.	11 Iris	47 Puls.	41 Nit-ac.	37 Nux-v.
45 Puls.	8 Phyt.	10 Merc.	43 Bar-c.	40 Kali-s.	37 Rhus-t.
44 Lach.	7 Arg-n.	10 Nit-ac.	42 Bell.	40 Sulph.	34 Arg-n.
42 Arg-n.	7 Aur-m.	9 Bell.	40 Arg-n.	37 Calc-f.	34 Bell.
42 Bar-c.	7 Calc-s.	9 Con.	40 Lach.	37 Sel.	34 Con.
37 Nux-v.	7 Calc-sil.	9 Rhus-t.	39 Sec.	35 Carc.	33 Alum.
37 Rhus-t.	7 Kali-i.	8 Puls.	36 Nux-v.	34 Con.	33 Hep.

Figure 2
Analysis of the Thiosinaminum Search by Category

Materia Medica for Thiosinaminum

From my own cases, I have compiled a small clinical materia medica for Thiosinaminum. Symptoms not currently in the repertory (Complete Repertory by Roger van Zandvoort) have been marked with an asterisk (*).

MIND
- Depressed.*
- Aversion to consolation.*
- Moody, alternating moods.*
- Dreams of being stuck and unable to move.*

GENERALITIES
- Allergies, seasonal.*

EARS
- Tinnitus.
- Otosclerosis.

ABDOMEN
- Pain secondary to scarring and adhesions.*

RECTUM
- Rectal stricture.

URINARY ORGANS
- Increased urination (frequency) at night.*

FEMALE GENITALIA
- PID.*
- Internal pelvic scarring.*

Final Comments

I believe Thiosinaminum is not just a small remedy. It is one that will require considerably more clinical use and shared experience over time before we can know if it has a significant application beyond the physical pathology of scarring. Even though these cases I have presented may suggest a few mental and emotional aspects of Thiosinaminum, there is obviously a great deal more to discover. I would, of course, be very interested to hear from anyone else who has experience with this remedy.

Guy Kokelenberg: I have had three Thiosinaminum cases. One was a patient with a keloid after burns with retraction of the arm, which is going better. The keloid has not disappeared, but the flexibility of the arm has improved. The second case was a person with reflux esophagitis with spasms and stricture of the esophagus, which was better after the remedy. The third one was even more agreeable. It was a case of Crohn's disease, which was better afterwards. There was a stricture of the intestine.

Audience: What potency did you use?

Guy Kokelenberg: I gave low potencies, but in Belgium we don't work very much with the "c" potencies. It was Korsakoff potencies, but low (6).

Riley: If you look at all of the old homeopathic literature concerning Thiosinaminum, it is difficult to understand exactly how they were using it. They are all talking about using grains of it, yet they are also talking about it being prepared homeopathically. I am not sure exactly where the crossover is, and I can't tell what dose they were using. However, it is quite clear to me they were talking about low potencies in daily doses.

Guy Kokelenberg: I have never understood the term "grains" as it is used in Boericke.

Audience: Maybe it was used as an injection.

Riley: Well, there is one mention of injections under the skin for scar formation.

Richard Hiltner: I think this is really good information. The mustard plant has some reputation in the treatment of cancer, and some research is being done in this area.

Also, in terms of seasonal allergies, we have Sinapis nigra, which is, of course, mustard. There may well be a relationship there, which would possibly explain why the sinuses were getting better.

Because there is such a close relationship between this remedy and Silica, I wonder if you or anyone else has found Silica to be helpful constitutionally in these cases or for backing up Thiosinaminum if it doesn't work in a particular case?

Riley: I haven't seen that. My initial bias was toward Natrum muriaticum in this regard, because I thought one of my cases needed Natrum muriaticum. I thought I would be able to find more of a relationship there, particularly with *the sense of depression and closedness. But at this point I would have to say I do not see a strong correlation with other remedies, although on the physical pathological level, certainly Silica is the closest.*

Marcia Neiswander: I am really grateful for this presentation. I gave Silica unsuccessfully to a patient recently. She was infertile following a second child. She moved to Israel, but this information will go in the mail to her when I return home. I have lost contact with her, but this may be the stuff that will help her to get pregnant.

Judyth Reichenberg-Ullman: What I noticed, on the mental and emotional levels in your cases, was that two people had dreams in which they felt trapped. They couldn't escape; they couldn't move. Did you ask the first person about this type of dream?

Riley: No. I didn't ask her.

Judyth Reichenberg-Ullman: I am thinking in terms of where the scarring came from. I have to wonder if and how this whole idea of scarring would present itself on the mental and emotional levels, prior to the physical scarring.

Riley: Yes. I think that is significant.

Murray Feldman: I would like to add to what Judyth has said, particularly as to the dreams of being stuck. When I look at the symptoms, in relationship to what you said about the scarring, the whole picture seems to be one of someone who is stuck in time, with a sense of hardening around him. And it may be due to emotional scars.

The fact that you used Natrum muriaticum in one case is very interesting. The remedy has senility, dementia, cataracts, premature old age, stiffness of the joints, ataxia, inelasticity of the skin. Looking at the "gestalt" aspect of the remedy, I found it fascinating that you mentioned the emotional scars in relationship to the physical scars, and the possible connection with Natrum muriaticum. There is very much a "stuck" element in the case. This is just something to think about in relationship to understanding the remedy more on a functional level, rather than on a strictly pathological level.

Riley: Thank you. So, in summary, let me reiterate. I would consider giving Thiosinaminum when I see the combination of depression or sadness with an aversion to consolation, in conjunction with significant physical scarring where the scarring is part of the chief complaint, or what you determine to be the chief complaint in a patient. It is especially relevant, in my experience, when you have pelvic scarring in women as a chief complaint.

And then the other two minor symptoms that seem to run through these cases—two minor "keynotes," for want of a better word—are seasonal allergies and increased urination at night.

References

Anschutz, E.P. (Ed.). 1990. *New, Old, and Forgotten Remedies.* Philadelphia: Boericke & Tafel.

Blackwood, Alexander L. 1923. *A Manual of Materia Medica, Therapeutics and Pharmacology with Clinical Index* (Rev. 2nd ed.). Philadelphia: Boericke & Tafel.

Boedler, Cornelia Richardson. Unpublished material.

Boericke, William. 1927. *Materia Medica with Repertory* (9th ed.). Philadelphia: Boericke & Tafel.

Clarke, John Henry. 1900. *A Dictionary of Materia Medica.* London: Homeopathic Publishing Company.

Grimmer. Unpublished material.

Ahmed Currim, MD, PhD

CLINICAL
EXPERIENCES
WITH
CARCINOSIN

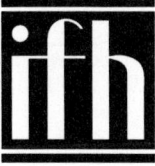

Ahmed Currim first encountered homeopathy in 1966, when he received a copy of Kent's Lectures on Homeopathic Philosophy *in the mail. He went on to complete his PhD and to teach college mathematics, but Kent's powerful words had "infected" him so profoundly that he eventually decided to pursue a new career. He graduated from the University of Brussels School of Medicine in 1979 and later completed his internship and residency in family practice in the United States. Dr. Currim has written the book,* Guide to Kent's Repertory, *which will soon be available. He also discovered Kent's repertory corrections while in India in 1980 and is currently working on a project to incorporate them into RADAR.*

Introductory Comments

I feel privileged indeed to be here in front of so many wonderful prescribers. I will try to share with you my current understanding of Carcinosin and how I arrived at it. Incidently, I have brought with me today a copy of Kent's *Lectures on Homeopathic Philosophy*. I received this particular copy on January 31, 1966, while I was a graduate student relaxing before a final exam the next day in mathematics, a subject of which I was very fond. Kent's lectures touched me very deeply then, and the "infection" never left me.

This book, which came from India, has been rebound twice. I have read it many times. It was Kent's inspiration that really changed my life. It made such a profound impression upon me. It changed me both professionally and personally. And it made me see deeper into life, into things I had learned from India, into yogic and Vedic philosophy, and into the unity of man.

Kent has been like a father to me. Whenever I feel upset and depressed I read Kent and I return to my life recharged. I would like to read to you the first paragraph of the last lecture, entitled "Difficult and Incurable Cases—Palliation." This paragraph always inspires me when I think I still have so far to go.

> While homeopathy itself is a perfect science, its truth is only partially known. The truth itself relates to the Divine, the knowledge relates to man. It will require a long time before physicians become genuine masters in this truth. In Switzerland, the children have been raised for centuries to know the knowledge that it is necessary to make watches perfectly, they have been raised, as it were, in the watch factories. Now,

when homeopathy is hundreds of years old, and little ones grow up into the knowledge of it and observe and practice it, our successors will acquire knowledge that we do not possess now. Things will grow brighter as minds are brought together and men think harmoniously. The more we keep together the better, and the more we think as one the better. It is a pity that differences should arise among us when we have so perfect a truth to bind us together.

I am so glad that we are here together, sharing the great truth that our masters, such as Hahnemann and Kent, have bequeathed to us.

The Carcinosin I use was prepared by Dora Schmidt-Nagel, the wife of Pierre Schmidt. She played a truly instrumental part in my life, providing assistance and inspiration. She encouraged me all through medical school in Brussels. She told me that she originally acquired the potencies from Foubister. I have a 200c, a 1M, a 10M, and a 50M. I have never used the 50M, but I have used the 200c, 1M, and 10M, and they have worked very well for me.

Case Number 1:
Polycystic Ovarian Disease

Female
Age 30

Initial Visit: April 23, 1992

She has been a hat designer for the last four years.

Dyspareunia. It started with excruciating pain on both sides of her abdomen. She was doubled over with pain for two to three hours.

Two days later she had pain after intercourse. She saw a gynecologist. He removed two labial warts. He also performed an ultrasound, which showed polycystic ovaries. One ovary had many cysts, and the other ovary had one large cyst and many smaller ones.

Other Test Results:
- Pap smear: Normal.
- Follicle-stimulating hormone/luteinizing hormone: Normal.

- Chlamydia, HPV screens: Negative.

Medications: Loestrin 21 1.5/30; takes very irregularly.

Herbs: Blessed thistle, black cohosh, dong quai, damiana.

Medical History:
- No mumps, measles, chicken pox, urinary tract infections, or vaginitis.
- Bronchitis.
- Tinea versicolor.
- Asthma until age 17.
- Cervicitis and cervical warts in 1987.
- Night fevers with sweats while living in Africa, about three to four times a year.
- Allergic to cats, dogs, and horses (raised in South Africa on a farm with horses).

Habits: Smokes one joint of marijuana daily.

Family History:

- Mother: Died of ovarian cancer at age 58; had many surgeries. Patient was born when mother had only one-half of an ovary left.

- Maternal Grandmother: May have had uterine cancer.

- Brother: Brain tumor.

Loves hot weather (3), even New York City summer heat. Hates cold weather.

Grinds her teeth while sleeping.

Menstruates two or three times a year; very irregular. No real PMS. Abdominal cramps. She started menstruating late, at around age 16; had one or two periods the first year. Fainted once in the early phase of one period. Her breasts developed at age 16.

She is very active in sports—biking, horseback riding, tennis. Has always been tall and gangly. Considered herself a tomboy.

Has not thought of having children.

Good appetite.

Desires chocolate (2), salt (2), spicy food (2), garlic (2) fruit (1), and spaghetti (1).

Averse to currants and raisins.

Has regular bowel movements. Diarrhea during menses.

"Claustrophobic" in a car if going down the road where there are lots of posts or trees. Her hands perspire if she is close to moving cars.

Has been with her husband for six years.

She has a difficult relationship with her father who travels a lot. "My father left my mother and moved in with another woman. He burdened me with his woes and the letters from this lover. I am the apple of his eye, but he is completely wrong in many cases. He overpowers me. I would like to say, 'Leave me alone.' One morning I was in tears and my husband told him to leave me alone. I have not seen him for two years."

"I am taking care of a friend dying with AIDS. I am very attached to him."

"I had a lot of pets and animals as a child."

"I think a lot of all my family."

Observation: She is a thin, 5-foot 5-inch woman with dark skin and dark hair. She is very pleasant.

Her husband confirms that she had pain one to two hours after coition early in 1992, that she had no pain for one to two weeks later, and that she has had major pain related to deep penetration over the last four months. He says she does not like sweet and sour foods but devours chocolate in binges. He adds that she does not have much female fat, that she exercises or does physical work daily, and that she is high-strung.

Analysis of Case Number 1

I used the following symptoms for the original repertorization:

- Sympathetic.

- Mildness.
- Menses irregular.
- Menses delayed in young girls, first menses.
- Diarrhea during menses.
- Menses late.
- Pain during intercourse.
- Warts, condyloma, external genitalia.
- Tumors, ovaries.
- Riding in wagon aggravates.

A straightforward repertorization showed Calcarea carbonica, Natrum muriaticum, Phosphorus, Sulphur, Lycopodium, and Sepia. I did not feel strongly about any of these remedies but thought Calcarea was the best fit.

Plan: Calcarea 01 LM (Helios), twice a day for seven days followed with 02 LM (Helios) twice a day for seven days.

Follow-Up on Case Number 1

May 15, 1992

Her dyspareunia is better. Less pain or no pain.

She is feeling pretty good.

Less lethargy.

She menstruated in early May. It lasted four days, and she used four tampons each day. Her breasts got bigger one week after the bleeding started, and they got sore on the lateral and superior aspects.

She still suffers from claustrophobia.

"My good friend is dying."

Good energy.

She gave up chocolate for Lent and then ate a lot of chocolate on Easter Sunday.

Eats a lot of garlic and salt.

Assessment: I could feel that the Calcarea had made only a superficial change, even though she was pleased to see improvement in her dyspareunia. So, I reconsidered the case along the following lines:

- Asthma in childhood.
- None of the usual childhood diseases.
- Strong history of cancer in the family.
- Brownish skin.
- Desire for chocolate.
- Sympathetic.

In addition, I had read somewhere that Carcinosin is known for its use in polycystic ovarian disease.

Plan: Carcinosin 200c (Schmidt-Nagel/Foubister), single dose.

October 6, 1992

"I gradually felt better and better. I was very aware of getting stomachaches. I have felt very good the last two months."

Her menses are normal. She had diarrhea during her last menses, but she was traveling. Her breast tenderness is gone.

The dyspareunia is gone.

"I still feel dizzy if things (poles) go by me fast. I cannot take rides. That has not improved."

She thinks she still grinds her teeth.

She has stopped designing hats and is selling Christmas ornaments.

She has a cold and sore throat and would like a remedy for the cold.

Assessment: Carcinosin is the correct remedy.

Plan: 1. Bryonia for her cold.
2. Carcinosin 200c, single dose, after the cold subsides.

January 29, 1993

She took the second dose of Carcinosin 200c at the end of 1992.

She saw her gynecologist on January 26. The ultrasound showed no ovarian cysts.

She is feeling very well despite only sleeping an average of four hours each night.

She is working very hard. Will be traveling to Kenya for eight to ten months.

She skipped a period in November 1992. Her last period was on December 20, 1992. She gets emotional before her period.

Assessment: The Carcinosin resolved the polycystic ovarian disease. (I ran the original repertorization on the RADAR program VES and it suggested Carcinosin.)

Plan: Carcinosin 1M (Schmidt-Nagel/Foubister), single dose, because she was going away for many months and was someone who would never take medicine regularly.

Case Number 2:
Chronic Depression

Female
Age 31

Initial Visit: February 19, 1993

She has suffered from depression for 12 or 13 years.

She is seeing a therapist. She was in a psychiatric hospital for one month in 1992. Can cope better since going to a network chiropractor.

She lives with her parents.

Feels a terrible darkness. Cannot get out of bed. Stays in bed for days at a time.

Has nervous breakdowns—screaming—and then collapses. Goes into a rage, and then sleeps.

Feels a terrible sadness.

Has a lot of anxiety and fear. Cannot leave home because she feels unsafe outside. Wants to stay isolated.

"I feel this poison in me. I have had no trauma. I had a sheltered upbringing. Then I went to college at age 18. It was like shell shock. I studied very hard. I lived in a dorm one year and then in an apartment. I had a lot of boyfriends but did not get serious. I was so withdrawn."

"When I get sad I love to eat, especially M & M's (chocolate). I am weight conscious. I go on eating binges and eat out of boredom—chips, hamburgers. Then I feel depressed and feel fat. If I gain two pounds I flip out. I get hungry at about 4 or 5 p.m. I love chocolate (3) and don't like hamburgers."

She loves to sleep. Has no problem sleeping. "It's the only time I have peace. I sleep from 10 p.m. until 5 a.m. I hate to be up and cannot wait to be back to sleep. I sleep in an unheated room but have a sheet, blanket, and two quilts. I sleep on my stomach with my face turned to my left side."

She dreams a lot about people and sharks. "I have a fear of sharks and going swimming in a pool by myself."

Her worst hour is 4 p.m. "I run at 4 p.m., and this releases anger, tension, and anxiety. I have a lot of anger because of this depression. The depression has resulted in a lot of lost opportunities in life. I am angry because people expect so much of me."

"I cannot concentrate. My photographic memory has diminished. I have no focus, passion, or interest. I am dead inside. I have less and less emotion for life, for people. I have no money. I live at home without privacy. I cannot live like an adult. I go home and I am by myself. I choose to be lonely. When my spirits are up I am fine but I do not commit to anything. I am not dependable. People cannot rely on me."

"I am suicidal. I think about it all the time. I would do it peacefully by cocaine, drink, or pills. I used to party in school and took cocaine to be social. One day I did it so much I almost died. Then, I swore I would never do it again."

Her menses are regular and "awful." She has tremendous cramps during menses. Cycles of bleeding a lot. "There are months when I am achy from head to toe." She is very depressed two to three days before menses. She feels anxious and irritable before menses. Her breasts swell and feel tender. Abdominal bloating.

Obsessed about her acne.

"I love my father and always wanted to please him."

(The patient's chiropractor, who referred her to me, had told me that the patient has no money, no job, and no social life. She stays at home and feels she is a total victim of her depression.)

Family History:
- Mother: Skin disease.
- Father: Gout.
- Maternal Grandmother: Cancerous polyp of the colon.
- Paternal Grandmother: Colon cancer.
- Maternal Grandfather: Heart disease.
- Paternal Grandfather: Heart disease; depression.

Analysis of Case Number 2

I found it confusing to unravel this case. Her highly volatile nature, together with the anger, depression, and anxiety that was worse from leaving the house, made me think of Ignatia. And seeing a notched tongue gave that remedy a good probability. But I did not see any history of recent grief and did not observe any sighing.

The menstrual symptoms brought several remedies to mind, especially Cimicifuga with the symptoms "terrible darkness" (Boger) and uterine cramping. And I obviously thought of Sepia. However, I felt that the following symptoms were the essence of the case:

- Family history of cancer.

- Conscientiousness or fastidiousness (about weight and acne).

- Craving for chocolate.

- Suicidal.

- Symptoms suggesting Sepia, Natrum muriaticum, and Ignatia without clear indications. (See Foubister's notes on remedies related to Carcinosin.)

Plan: One pellet of Carcinosin 200c (Schmidt-Nagel/Foubister), dissolved in one ounce of distilled water, ten drops every morning and evening for three days.

Follow-Up on Case Number 2

March 8, 1993

Telephone consultation.

She is feeling better overall.

Her concentration is better.

Plan: Wait.

May 2, 1993

Telephone consultation with her mother.

She is doing great.

She has moved out of the house, has a good job, and has a boyfriend.

"Her life has totally changed since she came to you. She is a manager in a country market."

August 17, 1993

"Same old stuff. I feel irritability running through my body. I feel fat, like I weigh 1,000 pounds. Everything sets me off. I am very sensitive and compulsive. If someone upsets me, I go crazy."

She gets very sick before her menses. Cramps in her uterus; better from heat and pressure. Lower backache and nausea. Headache; worse before, during, and after menses. Aching, flu-like symptoms around menses. Irritable before menses; breasts and neck feel puffy.

Suffers from motion sickness. Cannot read on a train.

Plan: Carcinosin 200c, in water, twice a day for three to four days.

August 30, 1993

Telephone consultation.

Her menses came on August 24 and is now ending. It is not as bad as before. The cramps are much better, the flow is less heavy, the back pain is much better, and the nausea and motion sickness are gone. She had only one day of flu-like symptoms.

She has panic attacks and sadness in the morning on waking.

She started running, which makes her feel better.

Impatient.

Her relations with her boyfriend are better.

Plan: 1. Wait.
2. Consider Ignatia, Sepia, Kali carbonicum, or Pulsatilla.

December 8, 1993

"I can be with my boyfriend or with a million people and still feel depressed, but I tune it out now and cannot be bothered. I love chocolate as much as before."

Her periods are "devastating, terrible." Two days of heavy flow (ten tampons); three days of spotting. Her back aches a lot one day before menses and two days during the flow. Her vagina feels sore and she urinates frequently during menses. She has a flu-like feeling, headache, and cramps before menses, but sometimes she is fine. No breast tenderness before menses. Very depressed before, during, and after menses. Stayed in bed on December 6 and 7, crying all day. "It was black. I thought I would go to the hospital. I dread my period. Sometimes I feel I have ovarian cancer."

"I need sun, a warm room."

"I feel I have a sinus condition."

She craves salt and chocolate.

"My boyfriend is good to me. He is the only reason I get out of bed. I love him and would marry him. I express love for him verbally, physically. It is a two-way relationship. We cannot do enough for each other. I feel I have someone who's worth fighting this illness for. It is not just sex, but showing emotion. He brings out a lot in me."

"I have to have a ton of ice in all my drinks. I love ice cream."

She is afraid of losing the people she loves, of suffering, of losing her own family. "That is why I do not like to get close to people. I feel it is hard enough to lose my family some day. So, if I marry and have children, I will have to worry about them dying." She is afraid of intruders and will not sleep alone in a house. She used to be deathly afraid of thunderstorms, but now it has diminished to about 40 percent of what it was. She could never sleep alone when she was young. She was afraid of the dark.

"When I was seven years old I had these depressions. I do not think I will ever be cured."

Assessment: This patient is not cured despite a very deep-acting remedy. Although she is much better, I wonder if my initial case taking was flawed. I did not get all these symptoms then. These new symptoms point to Phosphorus.

Plan: Phosphorus 200c, in water, twice a day for three days.

December 14, 1993

No change.

"I am very, very depressed. Unless you help me, I will have to take antidepressants."

Assessment: Carcinosin is the correct remedy. "You shall not change the remedy even though it would be impossible for you, at this date, from the present symptoms to select that remedy" (Kent, *Lectures on Homeopathic Philosophy*, lecture XXXVI, paragraph 11).

Plan: Carcinosin 1M (Schmidt-Nagel/Foubister), one pellet in one ounce of water, shake and take ten drops for three days.

January 5, 1994

Telephone consultation.

The depression lifted slowly but surely.

"I am feeling well."

March 14, 1994

Telephone consultation.

Her chronic depression is much better.

She gets depressed two days before menses and also has flu-like symptoms, but these symptoms are gone when the bleeding starts. Her relationship with her boyfriend is very good.

Panic attacks are better.

Plan: Wait.

Long-Term Follow-Up

She is doing well. She had another relapse. I gave her Ignatia, and she was better for two weeks. Then, I gave her Carcinosin 10M. Now she is really doing well. One lesson I learned from this case is that it is easy to mistake Carcinosin for Phosphorus or Ignatia.

Case Number 3:
Ulcerative Colitis

Female
Age 39

Initial Visit: December 4, 1990

She is 5 feet, 5 inches, and weighs 120 pounds.

She has five to six stools a day.

Current Medications:

- Prednisone, 30 mg per day.

- Robinul, 1 mg three times a day to prevent peptic ulcer from taking the Prednisone.

- Asulfadine, 500 mg four times a day.

- Xanax, as needed.

- Lomotil, as needed.

She started her menses at age 13½.

She started to have abdominal pain at age 14½; the pain extended toward her left kidney. She was starting high school at the time.

She is very conscientious—good student, good eater.

The pain would get worse while she was in school, and she would have to go home.

An upper GI series was done. Diagnosed as an irritable bowel.

She met her husband when she was 16; they married three years later.

"He went to Vietnam six weeks after our wedding. I was very worried about him getting killed. But I didn't have any stomach problems. I was watching my weight; skipped lunch and breakfast. I thought I was too heavy at 118 pounds. I wrote my husband every day. I was (and still am) very devoted to him."

She gave birth to a daughter. It was a good pregnancy. She had morning sickness, but would feel better after eating an egg and toast. Given Bendictine.

A year later she had a bad pregnancy. Her father died of a heart attack in her first month of pregnancy. He had colon cancer. She had bleeding (staining) for three months during the pregnancy.

They moved from Brooklyn to the Bronx to help her mother. "I was her sole support."

At 5½ months of pregnancy, she had uterine contractions and almost lost the baby. She was treated with an alcohol drip and bed rest. The alcohol treatment produced nausea and hunger. She gained 40 pounds during the pregnancy. Her son was born two weeks early, weighing 7 pounds.

Two years later her brother got lung cancer at age 33 and died. He was a smoker and a gambler. "I was devastated. We moved to Maryland in the middle of this. I was torn. I did not want to leave my mother, yet I had to go with my husband. In Maryland I felt disoriented, depressed, could not eat, could not take care of my kids, could not concentrate or read the paper. At the dining table I felt I was not really there. I was jittery. I wanted my husband while he was at work. I could not sleep. I would wake up at night. I could not cry. My mother came to take care of me. I saw a psychiatrist; took antidepressants. After five weeks, I cried."

"I had a fear of being alone, a fear that something would happen to my husband when he came home late."

"When I was 11 years old my mother would visit neighbors and I would watch her to make sure she got into the house next door and that nothing happened to her."

"When I was 10 to 12 years old I used to stay with a 60-year-old aunt. I was afraid my mother would not pick me up, that something would happen to her."

"I did not like to be left alone with my grandmother. My mother would lie to me and say she was going to the store and would go out Saturday nights."

She is afraid of airplanes and elevators.

"I like my house organized, and like to be home even if I am alone."

In the year after her brother's death she became pregnant again. Suffered from constipation, hemorrhoids, and a lot of pressure in her uterus during the pregnancy.

After the birth of a son, she had constant diarrhea for two weeks. She was put on a bland diet without milk. Then, she had blood in her stool. Her gastroenterologist diagnosed ulcerative colitis and found that one-third of her colon was diseased.

Desires chocolate (2), salt (2), chicken skin (2), and steak fat.

She did not have a period one month. Bloating and breast swelling before menses.

Analysis of Case Number 3

The main components of the case are ulcerative colitis, grief over the death of her father from cancer, and lots of medications.

I could not clearly see a remedy; however, the grief, fear of abandonment, gentle nature, and PMS symptoms made me choose Pulsatilla. Yet, I felt uneasy about this prescription. She was cold-blooded and liked fats. But I consoled myself that, given all her medications, this was my best choice and I would try to decrease her medications.

Plan: Pulsatilla 12c, one pellet dissolved in water to take by the plussing method.

Follow-Up on Case Number 3

December 18, 1990

She is feeling better.

Her diarrhea is reduced to two or three times a day.

Plan: Pulsatilla 01/LM (Helios), twice a day.

January 8, 1991

She feels better.

She was able to stop taking the Xanax, Lomotil, Asulfadine, and Robinul. Is still taking prednisone, 10 mg every day.

She stopped taking Pulsatilla 01 on her own. Since then, her stools are more frequent but are formed.

Plan: Pulsatilla 02/LM (Helios), twice a day.

January 30, 1991, through April 19, 1992

I gave this patient increasing potencies of Pulsatilla, from 03/LM to 18/LM (Helios), with gradual improvement.

She stopped all allopathic medication.

Large boils that she had in the past returned; they broke out on the left side of her neck and on her right mandible.

She has PMS, with sore breasts and bloating.

Her energy was low at 3 p.m. for about an hour or less.

Feels tired in the evening.

Gained ten pounds.

Not hungry for breakfast.

Gets an early morning urging for stool; the stool is mixed with blood and pus. Has a normal stool one hour later.

Dislikes cold weather.

Feels nauseated and queasy; better after eating and open air.

As a child, she suffered from carsickness on long trips.

Desires cold drinks.

Low back pain (an old symptom).

The nausea disappeared during this 15-month period.

Her hands are numb.

She gets hungrier before menses. Craves sweets and chocolate four to five days before menses, but the time decreased to only one day before menses as she continued her treatment.

Her chronic sinusitis returned, and then it improved somewhat.

Craves steak and fat.

Her symptoms are aggravated from cheese and tomatoes, which give diarrhea.

A grade II colonoscopy in November 1991 showed the following:

Chronic inflammation.

Infiltration of colonic mucosa with lymphocytes, plasma cells, eosinophils.

Some areas of cryptitis.

Infiltration of neutrophils.

No dysplasia.

April 20, 1992

She has generally improved.

She has only three stools a day.

She is able to travel and do far more than before.

She spoke of all the chocolate and spicy food she had eaten during Easter and mentioned how much she suffered with anxiety when members of her family were away and not back on time.

Assessment: I based my prescription on the constant anxiety for her family, the sympathy, the strong history of cancer in the family, the desire for chocolate and spices, and the fact that she still had ulcerative colitis.

Plan: Carcinosin 200c (Schmidt-Nagel/Foubister), single dose.

April 30, 1992

Telephone consultation.

Her appetite has increased.

She feels more energy and is much better emotionally.

Plan: Carcinosin 200c, only if symptoms return.

July 7, 1992

She had taken one dose of Carcinosin 200c in May.

She is doing well.

No diarrhea, except for two weeks ago, and it lasted five days. It started after she ate ice cream.

She cannot eat cold cuts.

Good energy.

The tiredness at 10 p.m. is gone.

"I am so much better. It's the best I have been."

The desire for chocolate has lessened.

The anxiety for her family members is less. "If my teenage daughter is not back by 12:30 a.m., I rationalize that she would call if there was a problem."

"Anxiety really aggravates my condition. During Christmas and summer if I overextend myself (with my kids) I get diarrhea."

Plan: Carcinosin 1M (Schmidt-Nagel/Foubister), single dose.

January 25, 1993

She is doing well.

She has occasional loose bowel movements and cramping. No blood.

Her anxiety is better.

Her craving for chocolate and ice cream has lessened.

She has hot flashes at night.

No menses since December 1992. (Menopause?)

Recent breast exam and Pap smear are normal.

Physical Examination: I noted a café au lait spot on her right clavicle during the breast examination.

Plan: Carcinosin 1M, single dose.

March 16, 1993

On February 10 she had a colonoscopy with multiple biopsies. They showed focal mild epithelial dysplasia in two places of the colon (hyperchromasia and nuclear enlargement). The biopsies were reviewed by a second hospital, which confirmed the microscopic findings.

Assessment: She was told by the gastroenterologist that she must be watched very carefully and may need to have a hemicolectomy. Yet, she said she has never felt better. She has no more diarrhea or bleeding, and her bowels are normal in every way.

Plan: Carcinosin 1M, single dose.

June 15, 1993

She had an episode of frequent bowel movements for two days, with some mucus, gas, and a little blood.

She is anxious about her daughter who works as a waitress until 1 a.m. and is a lifeguard during the day.

Craves chocolate once in a while and before menses.

Gets dizzy and a sour stomach after drinking coffee.

Assessment: Slight relapse.

Plan: Carcinosin 10M (Schmidt-Nagel/Foubister), single dose.

July 30, 1993

She had a big party for her daughter's graduation. Since then she has had some diarrhea; three to four bowel movements a day.

She still has anxiety over her children; waits up for them, even until 1:30 a.m., and then feels her stomach acting up.

Less craving for sweets.

"My kids call me a neat freak."

Assessment: Acute diarrhea.

Plan: Arsenicum 320c, in water, morning and evening for three days.

March 20, 1994

She is doing very well.

On February 23, she had another colonoscopy with biopsies. Colonoscopy results were as follows:

Normal cecum.

Multiple discrete areas of erythema, edema, mild friability, and in some cases ulcerations throughout the colon.

No polyps or exophytic lesions.

Normal right colon.

Normal-appearing hepatic flexure, transverse colon, and splenic flexure, except as mentioned above.

Mild to moderate atrophy and a haustral appearance to most of the transverse, left, and sigmoid colon.

Small hemorrhoids identified in rectum.

In the biopsies, seven specimens were taken from different sites in the colon. Those sections of the right colon are unremarkable. Beginning with the biopsies at 100 cm, the results were as follows:

Chronic active inflammatory disease throughout the remaining biopsies.

Acute cryptitis, basal plasmacytes, increased eosinophils with alterations in crypt architecture.

Paneth cell metaplasia in a number of the biopsies.

Prominent splaying of the muscularis mucosae.

No definite dysplasia.

Assessment: She is decidedly better. The dysplasia seems to be gone. However, this could be a pattern of the ulcerative colitis, namely dysplasia is seen on occasion and disappears on occasion. The patient needs periodic follow-up, but we are grateful to homeopathy for her current wonderful well-being. I have to wonder if the Arsenicum had any beneficial effect.

Plan: Follow-up soon.

June 1, 1994

"I have never felt so well in my life. I am really doing well."

Assessment: This woman has done very well indeed. I don't think she is going to have any more ulcerative colitis, nor will she need a colectomy. Perhaps I am biased, but I think this woman is cured. She feels so well mentally and emotionally. She is in excellent shape physically. Her sense of well-being from homeopathic treatment is evidenced by the many other patients she has referred to me.

Case Number 4:
No Appetite Control

This is the case of a very obese woman. She weighed about 260 pounds and was completely unable to control her appetite.

I relied on a few of the major keynote symptoms in order to prescribe, especially a strong family history of cancer and a tremendous craving for chocolate.

Plan: Carcinosin 200c, twice a day for three days.

This woman is now doing absolutely wonderfully. Her appetite is under control, and her weight is coming down. Her menstrual periods, which were also a problem, are better. She is progressing remarkably well.

Case Number 5:
A Psychic Propensity

Female
Age 55

This case is a rather unusual one. I might even call it weird. The prescription itself was not very difficult. The unusual aspect of the case was the psychic propensity of the patient, especially the experience she reported on follow-up.

Initial Visit

She came to me with a chronic gastritis that had been treated since 1976 by Mylanta. The problem had begun six months after her father died and had been symptomatic intermittently ever since then. The most recent flare-up was in March 1993 when her mother died.

"In the past four years my mother and I had bonded together and had cleared out our old issues. I know the 'baby' inside of me is still healing the pieces that I did not heal with her before she died. I have a wonderful shrink and a good support group."

"My husband is emotionally abusive, because he was physically and emotionally abused by his parents. I want to get strong enough to leave him. I don't want my husband to find out how I really feel about him until I am strong enough to leave him."

She had one daughter from her first marriage. She married at age 19 and had her daughter at age 25. Her first husband left her for another woman when the daughter was seven. She has been married to her second husband for five years. "For five years he has been abusive, but I felt it was my fault."

"My stomach aches after I eat. I have burning in my chest. I am always hungry. I am fine after I eat, but I feel hungry. I like dark chocolate, chocolate-covered halvah, and ice cream with chocolate. I also like barbecued hot dogs. I can't stand fat, lima beans, kidney, and licorice."

"I am a Virgo. I love order. I love neatness. I love cleanliness. My husband is a slob. I married him because he was great sexually and good in his profession."

"My mother abandoned me emotionally." (Carcinosin has been added for "Forsaken feeling" in both the Synthesis and the Complete Repertory.)

"My father sexually abused me—incest. He took showers with me. He never put the penis inside, but he did inappropriate touching. He would walk naked in front of me and put it all around my face. I was very angry at him for a long time. I later realized it was not all his fault and that my mother was not protecting me."

She had psychic experiences after her father's death. It was as if he came back and made amends, a healing experience. She described other psychic experiences, including one in which she woke in the night and saw her ex-husband standing there, smirking yet in a desperate state, asking her to pray for him. She later found out that his second wife and his father had both died, and he was left with a seven-year-old daughter from the second marriage. This was at a time when she was trying to get him to pay child support.

She goes to sleep at midnight to 2 a.m. and gets up at 9 or 10 a.m. She never sleeps on her abdomen, always on the back or on the side. She throws off the covers. Her feet are cold, and she sometimes wears socks in bed.

She used to love the warm and hate the cold. Now she loves the cold and hates the warm.

Likes the open air.

Loves bad weather and storms. She says they are "gorgeous."

Has hay fever from August until October.

Her periods were regular until age 35. She used to always be able to feel when her periods were going to come. She has fibroids. Has bloating three to four days before her period.

She is very sympathetic.

Family history of cancer, diabetes, and heart disease.

Assessment: I saw the same pattern in this case: the family history, a very sympathetic woman, the craving for chocolate, a history of chronic gastritis, and so on.

Plan: Carcinosin 1M (Schmidt-Nagel), single dose.

Follow-Up

Ten days later a strange thing happened. She called me and said, "I had a psychic experience. As soon as I left your office, I saw a beautiful thing—those little pellets that you put on my tongue were all churning around like white stars inside of me."

And then she said, "Later on, I saw myself on an operating table surrounded by seven hooded people. I peaked under the hoods and I saw my two grandfathers, my two grandmothers, my favorite aunt, and my parents. They were using instruments and were pulling out things that weren't supposed to be in my body. I felt this happening several times throughout the day."

She came back on follow-up feeling absolutely well. She had never before felt so well. Later, an old chronic sinusitis came back and resolved without treatment. I have continued to wait. Nothing else has been prescribed. She continues to do well in all respects.

I don't quite know what to make of the experiences she reported after the remedy. I can only say that I wrote it all down as she was telling it to me. She definitely appears to have benefitted greatly from the remedy. I am learning new things from this remedy, things I never before knew were possible.

A Summary of Carcinosin

The following summary of Carcinosin will often prove helpful in prescribing. The new repertory, Synthesis, compiled by Frederick Schroyens, MD, of Belgium has all of these symptoms (and many hundreds more). Furthermore, this repertory gives the sources. Many of the symptoms were given by the originator, Dr. D.M. Foubister (Fb), in the article, "The Carcinosin Drug-Picture" (*British Homeopathic Journal*, July 1958, Vol. XLVII, No. 3). To these were added others by Pierre Schmidt (St) and George Vithoulkas (Vh).

1. Fastidious, more than Arsenicum. This symptom was first given by Vithoulkas. States of anxiety, fears. Perfectionist, even more than Arsenicum. Perfection is a principle.

2. Anticipation (fears), ailments from. Fear of cancer, of being alone, of the dark (Case Number 2—December 8, 1993; Case Number 3—December 4, 1990), of health, of exams. Hypochondriasis (St).

3. Conscientious about trifles (Candagabe, Eugenio). LOYALTY. DUTY AT ALL COSTS, even to themselves (Fb)(Case Number 2—February 19, 1993).

4. Very sympathetic (Case Number 3—December 4, 1990).

5. Desires to travel as long as the strength is good (Vh). (This is the psoric side of the cancer miasm.)

6. Likes thunder, lightning (St). Also fears thunderstorms (Case Number 2—December 8, 1993). Can mislead you to give Phosphorus, as I did. So, watch out for this.

7. Offended very easily (St).

8. Has done so much, yet is trampled on and still does more.

9. Sensitive to reprimand (Julius Mezger). Children who have a history of many reprimands.

10. Repression, self-imposed. Doesn't cry easily. Keeps it within (Tinus Smits). Doesn't want to upset others. Must not be seen tired. Must not grumble.

11. Does not want consolation. Worse from consolation (Andre Julian).

12. Needs stimulation. Loves chocolate, even if sick after chocolates (St). Similar to Argentum nitricum, Sepia, and others.

13. Sleeps on abdomen (St) (Case Number 2—February 19, 1993). Compare with Ignatia, Medorrhinum, Pulsatilla, and others.

14. Insomnia (especially children). This is the syphilitic part of the cancer miasm (St) (Case Number 3—December 4, 1990).

15. Asthma in children (Case Number 1).

16. Anxiety for the welfare of family (Case Number 2—December 8, 1993; Case Number 3—December 4, 1990, and throughout the case). May make one think of Phosphorus and Arsenicum.

17. Multiple moles (Boericke; repertory).

18. Blue sclerotica. This is the syphilitic part of the cancer miasm, seen in osteogenesis imperfecta (Fb).

Currim: I have never seen this symptom of blue sclerae in Carcinosin cases.

Tinus Smits: It is almost always there. I have seen it in nearly all of my Carcinosin patients. I think the problem is that we don't look correctly at the sclerae. I have rarely seen a true Carcinosin case with white sclerae. There is always a blue halo.

Jonathan Shore: It is not prominent—very subtle. It is quite common, but you have to look. The white has a bluish tinge to it.

Currim: Thank you. I will look for it.

19. Café au lait skin, or spots (Fb) (Case Number 1—brownish skin; Case Number 3—January 25, 1993).

20. Tendency to occipital headaches. Similar to Lachesis.

21. History of repetitive childhood diseases—whooping cough, pneumonia, fevers, enlarged glands—or no childhood diseases (Case Number 1), or childhood diseases that appear in adults. (This last syndrome is well known in immune-suppressed patients and should alert us to the use of this nosode even in such acute diseases).

22. Never well since DPT shots, especially after pertussis vaccine. (See remarks in Foubister's original article regarding whooping cough and Carcinosin.) Is the increased incidence of breast cancer related to DPT shots?

23. Family history of cancer. Any family history of cancer should alert us to the need for this nosode, which will be needed at some point in the case. Also, family history of diabetes, tuberculosis, pernicious anemia, syphilis.

24. Resembles Pulsatilla, but they desire warm weather and warm rooms.

25. Resembles the intense anxiety or suppressed anger of Ignatia.

26. Relationships to the other remedies (see Foubister's article). Similar to Arsenicum, Phosphorus, Pulsatilla, Ignatia, Natrum muriaticum, Calcarea phosphorica, Sepia, Tuberculinum, Medorrhinum, Syphilinum, and Sulphur.

Judyth Reichenberg-Ullman: I have used Carcinosin frequently, mostly because of Jonathan Shore's lectures. [Editors' Note: See Dr. Shore's presentation in the 1989 IFH case conference proceedings.] *I understand that it is made from breast cancer. I noticed that in your three cases there was breast tenderness, but in most of the Carcinosin cases I have had there was much more ovarian pain. That has always seemed very curious to me. I would think there would be more of an affinity with the breast. Also, it doesn't make sense to me, with what we know about Carcinosin, that the patients should be averse to consolation.*

Currim: The aversion to consolation came out in one of these cases. I found this symptom in the Synthesis, where the reference for "consolation aggravates" is from Andre Julian. [Editors' Note: The Complete Repertory includes a reference to Carcinosin from Pierre Schmidt under "consolation aggravates." Carcinosin is also listed under "consolation ameliorates," with a reference from James Stephenson.] *It is true that these people are very sympathetic toward others. The feeling I have is that they want to do everything for the world, but if somebody comes to give them consolation or to take care of their illness or to give them help, they say, "I'm all right. I don't need it. I'm okay. Keep working. No problem." That is the kind of aversion to consolation that I have seen in Carcinosin. They are very hard workers. It is almost as if they are a little ashamed to show their weakness. They are stoic.*

As for the second question, about affinity for the breast and the ovarian tenderness, I can only say that several of my Carcinosin patients experienced PMS with breast tenderness.

Helene Schwartzenberger: Would a history of craving for chocolate in the lifetime of the patient suffice for prescribing Carcinosin, or does it have to be a current craving in order to give the remedy?

Currim: In most of my cases the craving for chocolate was a chronic one, since they were young, not one of recent appearance.

Helene Schwartzenberger: Have you ever seen any flu-like symptoms as an aggravation from taking Carcinosin?

Currim: I can't really confirm that. I will have to pay more attention to see if that occurs.

Jonathan Shore: I have an incidental comment about something that has interested me. I have been unable to get any pharmacy to identify the source of the remedy. When I was in Germany, I asked someone to call Schmidt-Nagel. They said, "Well, Madame Schmidt died and she never kept any records." I have not yet found a pharmacy that says it knows the source of this remedy. It is not that it doesn't work. (audience laughter)

Currim: *Well, I did know Madame Schmidt. Thanks to her, I became a doctor. In 1973, I visited her. She told me that Foubister provided the Carcinosin potencies that she gave me and that he made the remedy from a tissue sample of a woman patient with breast cancer. However, Madame Schmidt did not know the exact nature or type of the breast cancer.*

Tinus Smits: *I think that Carcinosin is one of the great remedies in homeopathy, a remedy not well known and often not quite correctly prescribed. I have prescribed Carcinosin for approximately 400 patients, and I have summarized my experience in my book,* Practical Materia Medica for the Consulting Room. *Thank you for your beautiful cases.*

Currim: *Yes, I have been waiting for your book.*

Tinus Smits: *Perhaps I might talk a bit about my experience with this remedy. One important clinical symptom is frequent blinking of the eyelids—rapid movement of the eyelids. Another symptom is moles and warts, especially on the soles and the palms of the hands. That is typical for Carcinosin.*

The forsaken feeling is, I think, not a symptom of Carcinosin but of another remedy that follows after Carcinosin. I will talk about that remedy in my presentation on Sunday. [Editors' Note: See Dr. Smits' presentation on Saccharum officinale in this book.]

The aversion to consolation, in my experience, is not an important symptom for Carcinosin. The patient may have this symptom, but you cannot decide the prescription on this symptom.

Other symptoms are more important, for example, the fears. They are afraid of crowds, narrow places, high places, spiders, mice, and snakes. For a long time I asked Carcinosin patients about all the fears of animals. The three fears that came out most frequently were mice, spiders, and snakes. The most frequent was spiders. They also are afraid of getting cancer, failing in examinations, failing in general, the dark, thunderstorms, and strong windstorms.

Concerning the fastidiousness, I don't agree that Carcinosin is more fastidious than Arsenicum. The fastidiousness of Carcinosin is a special kind of fastidiousness. These people are fastidious in their work, in whatever they are performing, because of their insecurity and their desire to be perfect. So, whenever they do something and present it to other people, it must be perfect. They are fastidious because they can be criticized. They feel that they can be criticized for almost anything, so they must be perfect. But they can be very untidy in their home or their clothes. That is not like Arsenicum. Arsenicum people display a neurotic fastidiousness, and they are fastidious because of a general insecurity. For me, it is completely different.

With regard to the PMS and other symptoms before menses, Carcinosin can be exactly like Sepia. I think that Sepia is the remedy that is most confused with Carcinosin. Carcinosin can have swelling of the breasts and painful breasts before menses. It can have irritability, sadness, swelling of the abdomen, and back pain before menses; everything can be like Sepia before menses.

Another symptom I often find is a sensitivity to "horrible" things. I ask if there are some TV programs they cannot stand to watch, and often they say, "Oh, when there is killing and horrible things, I close my eyes or I change the program."

And then Carcinosin exhibits a desire for and a sensitivity to music, often weeping from music. Like Sepia, Carcinosin loves dancing and has a good feeling for rhythm.

Carcinosin can show a desire to read, and yet these people can have dyslexia. Most Carcinosin patients who do not like to read are dyslexic or have such bad concentration that they cannot read. That is an addition I made, "Impossible to read because of a difficulty with concentration."

Other symptoms include the desire to travel, as you noted already, and nausea during traveling. There is a love of nature, animals, and thunderstorms, but also the fear of thunderstorms.

Still, ailments from a difficult education and upbringing are the most important indications for this remedy. These ailments and some of their causes include a sensitivity to rudeness, long-term domination, excessive parental control, harsh upbringing, too much responsibility too early, sensitivity to reprimands, strong reprimands as a child, prolonged fright, long-lasting grief, and long-lasting unhappiness. I will stop there.

Currim: *Thank you very much for these additions. Some of the things you have said are in my summary, but you have given us some helpful additional information. And I think you have answered the question about consolation.*

Tinus Smits: *It is a very important remedy that is often overlooked. I have seen really beautiful cures with Carcinosin.*

In your second case, you waited until there was a falling back. I don't wait. I repeat the remedy much more frequently.

Currim: *I am happy to hear that. Yes. I felt I learned something in that second case.*

Karl Robinson, MD

HOMEOPATHY: WORKING IN THE SACRED SPACE

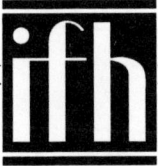

Karl Robinson received his BA from Yale University and his MD from Hahnemann University. After completing a residency in internal medicine at Harlem Hospital, he became interested in alternative medical therapies, eventually choosing homeopathy. Karl has studied homeopathy throughout the world, most recently in India with Rajan Sankaran, and is past editor of the Journal of the American Institute of Homeopathy. *He currently practices in Houston.*

Introduction: Homeopaths as Shamans— Divining the Patient's Myth

This is, I believe, a monumental decade for homeopathy. We are fortunate to be a part of it. So many changes are occurring so quickly. I have the feeling that some, or perhaps all, of us are moving along the path to becoming "shamans." As you know, so much in the homeopathic provings is interesting, unusual, and even weird— alluding to other realities, other worlds. But homeopathy is also a very logical "left brain" type of endeavor.

Speaking of shamanism, I went running this morning and just as I was leaving my motel, which is in a very urban area, a crow started vociferously cawing and then started swooping at me. I thought, "Ah, this is a message. I must be attuned to these things. If I continue on this path, I will be mugged." (audience laughter) So, I turned left and ran to the Space Needle. I hadn't planned to go there, but it was quite interesting. I ran all around the Space Needle and then returned. As I approached the motel, that same crow was there and it began swooping at me again.

I thought, "Well, it doesn't figure anymore. He is not warning me now. Now, he is just after me." (audience laughter) There were some street people sitting there, and they said, "Well, this crow probably has some young in a nest nearby." Who knows? It's extremely interesting. For any event, there is always the very reasonable explanation and then there is another possibility. The direction of my run was changed. Who can say which explanation is nearer the truth?

The initial homeopathic interview is, without doubt, a unique event. It is the one thing that cannot be taught very well. It can only be hinted and pointed at through various kinds of instruction. What happens between the homeopath and the patient within the confines of four walls is not an ordinary, sequential, or even reasonable occurrence. Within that space and that hour the principles governing ordinary human intercourse are suspended. If the patient has a desire to get better and if the homeopath has a desire to help the patient in that regard, then strange, nonsequential, nonlinear, and illogical events can and should begin to manifest.

In fact, the patient doesn't even have to wish to get well. Many children certainly don't wish to be in the homeopath's office! Some adults are there only to please a family member or a friend. So who or what actually gets them there at that particular moment? The higher self, the unseen "guides," the unconscious?

Something gets them there. We all know, even if we are beginning homeopaths, that extraordinary things can occur during the homeopathic interview. I have been teaching a nurse about homeopathy. She has been watching me take cases. Recently, she said to me, "I have been meaning to tell you. I had a kind of vision, a waking vision. Your office is a sacred place."

I was absolutely staggered by this comment. I said, "What do you mean?" She replied, "Well, it is a place where all these people feel free to talk about the extraordinary pain they are carrying. Within minutes, total strangers tell these amazing things. It is unbelievable."

I let that sink in. What an honor it is. What a space has been created that would allow people to speak, to feel, and to manifest in this way.

I call the initial interview the bewitching hour, the time when those subconscious, unconscious, and superconscious forces are given license to stir and perform their encoded dance. I say "encoded" because the patient's words, dreams, gestures, movements, and clothes tell a significant story. It is a story that begs to be decoded much as a fax machine receives bits of binary data and reconstructs them into written language.

Yet, the analogy is a poor one. Our patients don't even know the meaning of the story that they convey through their words or, more precisely, through their metaphors, together with their gestures, expressions, and movements. This is because their stories are their myth. It is this myth that homeopaths must read and decode into remedy. In that sense we are diviners. The initial homeopathic interview is filled with synchronicities—unrelated objects, events, words, and gestures that mysteriously come together and give meaning where before no meaning existed. This meaning is brand new and greater, much greater, than the previously unrelated parts.

The interview is like having a haystack in front of you. A golden needle lies inside the haystack. You absolutely know the needle is there. All you have to do is find it. That needle represents the remedy.

For all this to happen, the homeopath must provide the appropriate conditions. These conditions have little to do with furniture or pictures on the wall. It has much to do with the homeopath's manner, which must be kindly and totally "allowing." And it has everything to do with expectation. For some years now I have been trying to create (or you might say praying to create) conditions so that patients will reveal themselves and their remedy to me. Over the years these conditions have become more and more magical. I now expect that patients will perform—do their dance, say their myth—and I expect that I will be able to decode and find the remedy.

In this setting, even the mundane can become magical. What could be more mundane, for example, than the first minute when I ask for name, address, telephone number, and date of birth? Two months ago, here's what happened:

"What is your name?"

"Poppy."

"Poppy. That's an interesting name. Were you given that name or did you take it?"

"I gave it to myself."

"It's a flower, isn't it?"

"Yes. I've always liked it."

"What does it mean to you?"

"To me, it's special because it's strong yet flexible. It can bend and keep its center."

She went on to give a perfect description of Silica. Now, why did I comment on her name? I almost never comment on the patient's name, certainly never as I did with her. Somehow I divined that there was a clue there, so I pursued it.

The other day a young man came in. He was wearing a T-shirt that said, "Carpe Diem." I asked him what that meant, and he said, "seize the day."

Now, what sort of man would wear such a message? Someone who knows how to seize the day, seize the moment? A bold, buccaneer type? Hardly. This man was in his mid-thirties. He was unmarried, did not have a girlfriend, and was a virgin. When asked if he wished for a girlfriend, a wife, a sexual partner, he gave an ambiguous answer. His state was opposite to all that is bold and daring, to all that "seize the day" connotes.

But why does he own such a T-shirt? And why was he wearing it on *that* day in my office? I suggest that his shirt was part of that hour's synchronicity. It was a prop that his guiding forces led him to wear that day so that he could perform brilliantly in that half-hour drama. And, finally, it was necessary because it was part of his myth.

Now, let's explore three cases that illustrate these ideas.

Case Number 1:
Attention Deficit Disorder

Male
Age 9

Initial Visit: September 1992

The boy is brought to see me because he behaves in a disruptive way. He carries a presumptive diagnosis of attention deficit disorder. His mother reports that he has already been successfully treated with Belladonna for nightmares.

"I disrupt the class by humming and singing." His mother added that the reports from school mention that he gets out of his seat, stands on his chair, does not pay attention to the teacher, stares out the window for long periods, and spends such a long time sharpening his pencil that it gets noticed. "His teacher says he can't focus."

"He has no motivation," his mother says. "He doesn't like to work, and he refuses to do his homework. However, he does like to mow the grass and take out the trash. When he was younger he didn't like to do the usual kinds of things kids do with their hands, like blocks and puzzles."

He is not well organized and is messy. Despite these problems, his grades are in the 80s to 90s.

"I dislike school." Math is his favorite subject although he does not excel in it. His mother says that if he reads a math problem he can't do it. "For example, if he reads, 'If four chimps each have a baby how many babies are there?' he can't do it. But if he hears the problem he gets the answer." In the same vein, if he reads a paragraph he can't answer a question about it yet he can memorize the paragraph.

His favorite activities are playing soccer and swimming.

He has no anger to speak of. When he was younger he never shared his toys and was unfriendly to other children.

Desires pizza (2), oranges (1), fruit (1), and white bread.

Averse to meat, fat, fish, milk (2), cheese, chicken, and eggs (1).

He is fairly thirsty for cold water from the refrigerator.

"Whatever I fix, he eats," says his mother. "He has no strong cravings. But if the salad dressing spills over onto another food he won't eat it. He says it's 'contaminated.'"

Throughout the interview he is pleasant and cooperative but seems not fully present. The one exception is when he talks about his best friend. He seems quite animated as he speaks of the good times they have playing together, giving the impression that he and his buddy are very close. While he's talking his mother is looking at him in disbelief. "Aside from seeing that boy in church he has played with him only once in the whole year," she said.

He has a fascination with fires and can talk about them "for hours," according to his mother.

The pregnancy was uneventful except that his mother smoked cigarettes throughout. For the 11 years prior to the pregnancy she had used marijuana but stopped using it when she learned she was pregnant.

He is warm (2).

The interview ends with his mother saying in front of him, "He's strange."

"Why so?" I ask.

"Nothing excites him. He doesn't love any foods or sports."

Robinson: Where is the needle in the haystack here?

Barbara Newlon: What strikes me as strange is that there is something going on with this boy's sense of time. He spends a brief time with someone and feels they are close friends, and then he spends a long time sharpening his pencil and is oblivious. That struck me as strange, rare, and peculiar.

Robinson: Yes, that is interesting. Very good.

Barbara Newlon: Something is going on in his consciousness, in his memory. There is some kind of large gap in time and relationships.

Robinson: You are on the right track.

Durr Elmore: I would think of Cannabis indica for this case, especially because the mother smoked marijuana quite a bit before he was born. I think it is often indicated in a child like this, where one doesn't see the violence of some of the other hyperactive remedies yet the spaciness and the time distortion are prominent.

Robinson: Good. I gave Cannabis 1M to this boy.

Analysis of Case Number 1

I did not use specific rubrics to arrive at the prescription. What led me to the prescription were the boy's extreme spaciness—not his restlessness—coupled with the mother's use of marijuana for years prior to learning she was pregnant.

I believe the state of the parents beginning at conception and continuing through the pregnancy can determine the character and behavior of the child, sometimes for life. Although his mother quit marijuana as soon as she found out she was pregnant she was using it for at least the first three weeks, enough time to have an effect. Also, presumably it took her some months before she moved out of her cannabis-induced mental state.

Plan: Cannabis indica 1M, single dose.

Follow-Up on Case Number 1

October 1992

His mother had seen the boy's teacher the day before. The teacher was very pleased. She said, "It's hard to believe how much his work has improved in school. His ability to focus has improved unbelievably."

He is still disruptive in class—talking too much and singing and humming—but he is paying attention much better. Also, he is raising his hand to be called on more.

Both parents have noticed that he is doing his homework on his own without being reminded.

"You know, there really have been some remarkable changes," said his mother. "Only this week he said with enthusiasm, 'Boy, Mom, I really like this nacho cheese!'"

When I ask about his difficulties with reading math, his mother says he can now do it. In a recent quiz he got 19 out of 20 questions correct.

I note that as he sits in my office he is constantly kicking his legs and moving his shoulders up and down. He hums, and he rocks in the chair.

I ask the boy to step outside so that I can find out more about his mother's life before she became pregnant with him.

I say, "I want you to know the medicine your son received was homeopathic marijuana. Please tell me about the years you used marijuana."

At first she looks astonished and then shocked, and then she begins to weep. "I smoked a lot. I was a heavy user. But I stopped as soon as I knew I was pregnant. About that time we became Jehovah's Witnesses. A lot changed. But my husband was violent with me during the pregnancy. I figured he was having an affair. I was very suspicious."

"Did you have any bad experiences with marijuana?"

"Toward the end I got scared and hyper. But I always loved to smoke pot. I laughed a lot. I ate a lot. I enjoyed sex. It made me relaxed and dreamy."

Assessment: The remedy is acting. As I mentioned earlier, I did not use specific rubrics in the repertory to arrive at the prescription. However, if we look at the symptoms of the mother's state, we find they are all covered by Cannabis: anxiety (bold type), suspicious (bold), laughing (bold), as if in a dream (italics), appetite increased (bold), and sex desire increased (plain).

Plan: Wait.

February 1993

He is not completing about two homework assignments a week, suggesting some backsliding. However, the humming and singing in class have stopped. He is no longer standing in class when he's supposed to be sitting, but he is still talking too much in class. A report from the teacher suggests he is not as focused as he had been.

Desires oranges (3), eats two to four oranges a day; hot dogs with ketchup (1); bacon (1); and bologna (2). Chews ice (1).

Assessment: Although his food cravings were pointing to Medorrhinum, this did not affect my judgment. He had done too well on Cannabis indica to consider anything else. I decided to repeat the remedy because his concentration was waning slightly.

Plan: Cannabis indica 1M, single dose.

November 1993

He had done well all year until recently. He received an "A" for conduct even though he was associating with children who got "F." He is not completing all his assignments, despite reminders from his teacher. After taking the Cannabis in February he completed more assignments. His mother thinks his motivation has fallen off since then.

Observation: My impression of the boy 14 months after the first prescription is that he is a totally changed person. Now he is lighthearted with a sense of humor. He jokes with me. He seems alert, interested, and a hundred times more interactive and responsive. He had gone from a listless to a lively boy, from a spacy to an interested boy, and from a restless and agitated to an attentive and joyful boy.

Assessment: Because his mother felt his motivation had again fallen off, I repeated the remedy without expecting much more in the way of overall improvement.

Plan: Cannabis indica 1M, single dose.

> *Robinson: What is going on in this case? How does this happen? How does this nine-year-old boy end up manifesting a Cannabis state? He, himself, was not a Cannabis user. I would like to hear your theories. It is an absolutely theoretical question, of course. Be the shaman. Be the metaphysician. Be the geneticist (audience laughter).*
>
> *Richard Hiltner: Thinking in terms of Rajan Sankaran's methods, I wonder about the behavior of the father toward the mother during the pregnancy. This may have had something to do with it.*
>
> *Robinson: Okay, let's assume that is the case. How is it transmitted?*
>
> *Richard Hiltner: That I am not sure of. It seemed to be more of a violent behavior, usually not associated with Cannabis. But the suspiciousness and the other aspects you mentioned might have had an effect.*
>
> *Durr Elmore: The mother actually did a proving of Cannabis while she was still pregnant. She said she quit when she discovered she was pregnant. During those very impressionable and formative early weeks of pregnancy she was smoking marijuana daily, so the child was receiving both a physiological and an "etheric" influence.*
>
> *Robinson: Yes, but how is it transmitted?*
>
> *Durr Elmore: In a case like this, you could say that it was transmitted because she was actually taking it into her body. It would be trickier to explain if she had stopped a couple of months before becoming pregnant. Perhaps this could happen also. Then one would have to say it was some kind of genetic or "energetic" transmission. However, in this case the mother was actually taking it physiologically.*
>
> *Robinson: Okay, she is taking smoke into her lungs. The smoke goes across the alveoli, is picked up by the blood, circulates around, and goes into the fetus' blood supply. How is it transmitted?*

Durr Elmore: Through the blood.

Robinson: What actually goes on?

Durr Elmore: If the mother is under the influence of marijuana, then the baby is getting it through the blood and it is also affecting his brain.

Marcia Neiswander: It seems she was pregnant for several weeks before she discovered that she was pregnant. During that time she probably was still consuming the marijuana, so there was a window from the time that she conceived until the time that she stopped. Moreover, marijuana is bound in the fat cells. When you start to detoxify after use is stopped, a lot of marijuana comes out of the fat cells into the bloodstream. She, and therefore the fetus, may have had a much higher dose of Cannabis in the bloodstream because she had quit.

The other aspect that I find very interesting concerns how the father's aggression may have affected the mother. Battered women tend to withdraw emotionally, and they frequently can have a very distorted time sense that, by whatever mechanism, was transmitted to her son. He behaved like someone who is very distant in time from what is going on around him. Because of the abuse, his behavior took on a surreal, almost Fellini-esque, kind of reality.

Roger Morrison: I have been exposed to two cases, one of my own and one that I have seen, where children have required homeopathic Cannabis indica at a very young age. One, a case of grand mal seizures that was cured by Cannabis indica 10M, and one, a case of behavior disorder with symptoms similar to your case in which the mother never used Cannabis indica but the father had used it. In the first case, the father had not used Cannabis for a number of years yet the indicated homeopathic remedy was Cannabis indica. So, I don't think that we can make any claim that this is always transmitted physiologically in the body. We must assume that the mother somehow "imprints" onto the child, via some "dynamic" plane, the effects of the marijuana and, further, that these effects can even come from the father somehow.

Robinson: Okay, so what is your theory?

Roger Morrison: I don't have a theory. What I can say is that it is definitely not physiological.

Robinson: Go ahead and think. Tell me how it could be imprinted dynamically.

Morrison: I don't "think" (audience laughter).

Steve Olsen: I want to mention an experience I had with a woman patient. I treated her four-year-old son for extreme violent tendencies. He was also a chronic liar. The remedy that helped him was Morphinum, the homeopathic preparation of morphine. He has done quite well on Morphinum for two years now. Later, the mother told me she had used heroin for a year when she was 16 years old. She had her son in her late 20s. Her remedy was initially Hyoscyamus, and then she did very well on Ignatia. She never needed Morphinum, Opium, or any related remedy. So the Morphinum state was there and it got passed through, yet it wasn't because she manifested the state herself.

My theory is that the water in the body actually holds the information. Within the cytoplasm, it is the structure of water that holds the "memory." That is why the whole body can communicate so well with every cell, because it is communicating with all the information in the cytoplasm.

Tinus Smits: I also have a theory. I think that not only her physical body is intoxicated but also her etheric, astral, mental, and causal "bodies." We know from regression therapy that the child is in complete symbiosis with the mother. It doesn't have to be an actual physical intoxication. There is surely an intoxication on other levels. If a mother used drugs even ten years before, she can stay intoxicated on higher "energetic" levels and pass this kind of disturbance to a child she gives birth to later.

Judith Coates: I was at a seminar at Esalen with some of the world's most famous scientists. The seminar was about water. The majority of our planet is water, and the scientists were talking about the healing properties of water and the memory being in the water because of the cytoplasm. So, often when I give a remedy, I put it in water and then succus it, because I feel that the water retains the memory, or the "fingerprint" or "impression," that is in the remedy. I think water intensifies the remedy. My clients do not have such strong aggravations from remedies when I do this.

Janet Henneke: You invited comment along metaphysical lines, and I see the comments are becoming more and more metaphysical. So, I would like to add a comment. In terms of a central disturbance, such as Rajan Sankaran talks about, there is not just the central disturbance of the parents but there is also the central disturbance of the child who is coming into the physical body. In a sense, there is a sort of matching process that takes place on that "dynamic" level. We tend somehow to select parents who have a similar disturbance to our own, a disturbance that we are incarnating so that we can work on it.

Robinson: *Well, if all this speculation gets printed in the proceedings, this is going to kill homeopathy's reputation (audience laughter). I have a couple of other cases. Perhaps I should go on. The one thing I did not hear was the idea of "spiritus," that Cannabis the plant has a spirit, or deva, that jumps on to people. Just an idea...(audience laughter). I do think there is a subtle body phenomenon, as Tinus and others have said, but in this case it could also be explained physiologically. The mother did smoke for the first three weeks. Roger's experience suggests it is not physiological, so it is a question. I do believe that everything we do is numinous. We have to understand that.*

Case Number 2

Female
Age 74

Initial Visit: November 1993

The woman complains of pain in the right shoulder. In the last three weeks the pain has extended to the hand. A year earlier she had fallen and injured her right shoulder, hip, and ankle. The shoulder received the brunt of the fall. An x-ray of the shoulder was negative.

"It feels like hot needles, thousands of them, but only at night after I lie down."

The pain disturbs her sleep. Her friend, a lay homeopath, had given her Rhus toxicodendron 30c and then 200c. It had helped for a while.

Her right wrist, hand, and fingers appear swollen. There are no swollen or tender lymph nodes in the right axilla.

She also complains of numbness in the tips of her fingers that has been occurring for the past three weeks. "When I move my right fingers it causes a weird sensation in my left shoulder."

The burning pain is somewhat relieved by applying cold followed by hot. A warm cover on her right shoulder is soothing. The pain is worse from motion and from touch.

She has lost much strength in her right upper extremity and finds it hard to screw and unscrew jar lids.

The pain is so intense that it forces her out of bed at night.

When I ask about her character, the friend who brought her says with genuine admiration in her voice, "She is stable, responsible, and religious. She is exemplary."

When I ask if she prays, the patient replies, "All day long." She is a Jehovah's Witness. She is a perennial "Pioneer," one who spends 100 hours a month going door-to-door proselytizing. She has received Pioneer status every month for the past 12 years.

She takes care of a large house and manages over 40 rental properties. She follows a daily schedule and finds time to play the accordion.

She carries herself erect and has an air of nonegotistic pride about her.

Her husband died of cancer, and she fears her shoulder problem might be cancer.

Analysis of Case Number 2

Her mien suggests a person of substance, someone capable and confident. It is not an assumed demeanor, not an attitude, but a very deep part of her. It is as though she is of royal parentage. She takes her religious responsibilities very seriously, praying constantly and devoting 100 hours a month to spread the Word, in addition to the time she spends at the Kingdom Hall.

In Phatak's repertory, Aurum metallicum is the only remedy listed under Responsibility aggravates. We owe a lot to Phatak. It is well known that Aurum people are religious, and Aurum appears under the rubrics, Praying (bold) and Religious affections (italics).

Until the last few years Aurum was prescribed almost exclusively for depressed, usually suicidally depressed, individuals. Thanks to the pioneering work of Rajan Sankaran, this is no longer the case. Sankaran showed that most persons needing Aurum are not depressed but are very responsible, orderly, and religious. He covers Aurum nicely in his book, *The Spirit of Homeopathy*. Since studying with Sankaran I prescribe Aurum much more often and I find that many patients needing it are neither suicidal nor depressed. I find that they may have a history of depression.

The remedy is not known as a "shoulder medicine," nor is it known for numbness. It does appear under EXTREMITIES, Pain, paralytic, and EXTREMITIES, Pain, joints, paralytic. Note that her pain has rendered her nearly unable to unscrew lids from jars. Aurum also appears under GENERALITIES, Pain, burning, internally. However, I did not prescribe it on the basis of the physical symptoms. Even if I had found no repertory confirmation for the physical symptoms, I still would have prescribed Aurum.

Plan: Aurum metallicum 200c, single dose.

Follow-Up on Case Number 2

I never saw the patient in the office again. But her friend reported that she was sleeping through the night within two weeks after taking the remedy, as the pain lessened. Aurum metallicum 200c was repeated in December, and again once in early 1994 in the 1M potency. The shoulder has been virtually fine since.

Case Number 3

Female
Age 63

Initial Visit: September 1993

She is undergoing chemotherapy for a recurrence of metastatic breast cancer. She had a right radical mastectomy in 1983. The cancer returned two years ago. She received chemotherapy between August and December 1991. She has a pleural effusion of the right posterior lung; thoracentesis has been done twice, most recently in June 1993.

I told her at the outset that I did not treat cancer, but she hopes that I might help her with the side effects from the current chemotherapy. These include nausea, weakness, fatigue, and loss of appetite—all fairly extreme.

Her mother died of abdominal cancer when the patient was 13. "My mother never let the family know. It was a great shock to me. I didn't cry."

When she was 27 she bore her first child. "I was scared of the baby. I didn't know anything about babies. I had a complete nervous breakdown. I cut my wrists. I didn't want to take care of the baby." She was hospitalized for six weeks and received electroshock therapy. "The baby was nine months old before I loved him."

"I'm a nervous type of person, nervous inside." She becomes nervous in traffic.

"I'm afraid of dying." (She leaned to her right toward her husband and grabbed his hand.) "I'm so afraid."

Recently, she often says to her husband, "Hold me! I'm so afraid. I'm so afraid." (Her husband confirms this.) When she is most afraid she feels compelled to be with him.

She sleeps on her left and awakes twice during the night.

She is chilly (2); bothered by cold drafts (2).

She loves violent thunderstorms and the sun.

She relates a dream about her own funeral. "I was with my husband but unable to talk with him because he was on the way to my funeral."

Afraid of high places (2); pools, lakes, and oceans; dogs (1); and Siamese cats (1). "They are sneaky," she says of Siamese cats. She also is afraid of violence; is reluctant to watch TV news and refuses to see scary movies.

She reads the Bible daily for ten to fifteen minutes. She prays "on and off all day long."

Desires hamburgers (1), fried chicken (1), chicken-fried steak, Dr. Pepper (2), M & M's (2), ice cream (1), milk, cheese (1), sweets (2), bread, and eggs (2). She ate eggs five days a week until two years ago.

Afraid of insanity since starting the chemotherapy.

She gets short of breath going up only one flight of stairs since starting the chemotherapy.

> *Robinson: Any quick ideas on this? Remember, I am not trying to cure this woman's cancer. I am trying to give her a little relief.*

> *Audience: Cannabis indica, Arsenicum, Carcinosin.*

Robinson: Nancy, what do you think?

Nancy Herrick: Bismuth, because of the fear of death and the clinging.

Audience: Cinnamonum.

Robinson: You have me there. I don't know that remedy. So, I obviously didn't give it.

Bob Ullman: Stramonium.

Robinson: That is what I gave.

Tinus Smits: Another suggestion would be Electricitas, because she received electroshock therapy. I had a patient who was very depressed for more than 30 years after she received electric shocks for depression. I gave her some remedies that had no effect, and then I gave her Electricitas. After this remedy her depression went away marvelously. So, it is a remedy to think of in cases where there are problems after electrical shock.

Analysis of Case Number 3

This case is presented not as a cure, but to illustrate how homeopathy can be beneficial in situations where a cure may not be possible. I based the prescription on her extreme fearfulness. Her fear was out in the open, palpable, and very acute. She was so afraid that she actually grabbed on to her husband. In the repertories of Kent and Kunzli, see Clinging. She also has a strong fear of death, water, insanity, and dogs. Also, she cannot bear to be alone.

Persons needing Stramonium, whether for an acute condition or a chronic one, act as if they are in an acute emergency. Picture the night terrors of the child. The child wakes in the night and clings with an acute, wild-eyed terror. Then transpose that understanding onto any one, adult or otherwise, who is acting like that.

Stramonium types are clingy, either literally, as she was, or mentally and emotionally. They have a clingy, desperate sound in their voices and they leave desperate sounding messages on answering machines. They are among the clingiest of patients. Stramonium also is known for praying.

Plan: Stramonium 12c, daily.

Follow-Up on Case Number 3

Two Weeks Later

Her nausea has decreased by 50 percent; the fatigue and weakness have decreased by 75 percent; her appetite has improved by 50 percent; and her fears are "50 percent better at least." She had undergone another chemotherapy treatment since starting Stramonium.

When I ask if she is still clinging to her husband in fear and desperation, she said, "No. Not once!" She says she has no fear of dying.

She admits to liking potatoes (2).

Assessment: She is responding to Stramonium very well. Her underlying remedy appears to be Calcarea carbonica.

Plan: Calcarea carbonica 200c, single dose.

One Month Later

She had chemotherapy eight days ago.

No fears.

She is feeling a bit tired.

She is able to sleep on her right side now.

She has decided to forego the fifth and sixth chemotherapy treatments.

Assessment: She is doing well. She appears bright and cheerful. But she is tired.

Plan: Kali phosphoricum 200c, single dose.

One Month Later

"I'm doing fine." But she can't say whether the last remedy has acted.

Her physical energy is not good.

Plan: Kali phosphoricum 6x, three times a day.

One Month Later

Two weeks ago she began taking an androgenic hormone, which has caused fluid retention. Before she starting taking it she felt "quite well."

A CT scan showed no change in the pleural effusion of the right posterior lung.

She becomes short of breath if she walks too fast; it is much worse when walking upstairs or up an incline.

No mental symptoms.

Her thirst is low. Desires water at room temperature.

Averse to salty and spicy foods.

Assessment: She doesn't have any of the mental symptoms that led to the original Stramonium prescription. In fact, I couldn't find any symptoms to prescribe on. On the basis of her extreme good nature, the location of her lung pathology (right lower lung), and an intuitive hunch, I gave her Phosphorus. She began taking shark cartilage on her own.

Plan: Phosphorus 1M, single dose.

One Month Later (February 1994)

She is feeling better. She believes the shark cartilage is helping.

For two weeks after taking the Phosphorus she urinated copiously.

She is much less short of breath and is able to go up stairs more easily.

Physical Examination: Percussion and auscultation of the right posterior lung field indicates two to three inches of dullness, suggesting that the effusion has not diminished.

Assessment: The copious urination can hardly be explained by shark cartilage. Phosphorus produced the heavy urination and subsequent improvement in breathing. Because the increased urination had stopped after two weeks I gave her Phosphorus again.

Plan: Phosphorus 10M, single dose.

One Month Later (March 1994)

She is doing well.

The shortness of breath is still improving.

She had increased urination for about ten days following the last dose of Phosphorus. It decreased for about 12 days and then recently began to increase again.

Nocturia three to four times.

Physical Examination: The right posterior lung field is unchanged.

She is "a lot better" on stairs.

She takes Halotestin, one daily.

Plan: Phosphorus 50M, single dose.

> *Robinson: It is interesting to see how the mental and emotional symptoms were so useful in prescribing for the treatment of rather ordinary, albeit intense, physical symptoms subsequent to chemotherapy. So, we can never discount the mental symptoms. Homeopathy has moved through various philosophical phases. The Sankaran influence, which is currently on the wax, says that all illness is in the mind, which I believe. However, we have to take*

into account that brilliant presentation that David Riley gave on Thiosinaminum. That has to be interpolated, inserted, implanted into our understanding, because the remedies are vast.

Remedies work on all levels. They don't have to work just on the mental level. We know all too well that most of the people doing homeopathy in the world aren't practicing it in the "elite" way we are trying to practice. But they are all getting some results. The remedies are a lot more intricate and interesting than we know. It is important to understand that there is no one way to approach a case, that we can help people in many ways, and that it is no sin to help a person physically from time to time (Audience laughter).

Ahmed Currim: *I want to thank you, Karl, because you took me back to a time when I was an intern. I trembled when I had to see the patients in the hospital, and I have a "confession" to make. I was called at 5:45 in the morning for a man with metastatic lung cancer. The cancer had spread to the liver. His bilirubin was around 20. He was really as yellow as they come. He had been given morphine and also Demerol, 100 milligrams every one to two hours. It did not touch his pain.*

He was in real agony, so they called me to give him IV morphine because the nurse could not give it. They woke me up and told me a few symptoms. I was a bit of a rebel. I put three remedies into my pocket, Antimonium tartaricum, Arsenicum, and one other which I have forgotten. When I went to see him he was breathing at about 50 to 60 respirations per minute and his pulse rate could not be counted. His private nurse who was with him said she thought it was around 170 to 180.

*I still see him well in my memory. I remembered the article on euthanasia by Kent in his **Lesser Writings**, and I had always been touched by it. I looked at him and just asked him, "Mr. Smith, are you having pain?" He couldn't talk much but he looked at me and he begged me. The rubric, Begging, in Kent's repertory came into my mind. Two remedies are there. You struck one today, Stramonium, and I struck the other one at that time, and the remedy was Arsenicum.*

The nurse said, "What are you doing?" I said, "Go, run, get him oxygen." I pulled out the packet of Arsenicum from my pocket. I can still see the packet. I put a dose of 10M onto his tongue. I didn't have time to put it back in my pocket before he heaved a sigh and just shut his eyes. In about 45 seconds his heart rate had come down to where I could count it, somewhere around 100, and he passed away in complete peace. I cannot tell you how much this touched me. It was a profoundly deep experience, just by remembering this one rubric. One dose of 10M touched him and gave him full peace to go further on, whereas all the Demerol and all the morphine hadn't touched him for two days. It was as if I was called. God said, "Currim, come. Take care of this and then get out." I had to run off because I had to attend to somebody else.

I thought I would share this, because your Stramonium case evoked this in me. In fact, I see in retrospect I missed Stramonium in another dying patient. I gave Arsenicum. It was the same clinging, and you showed me that I should have given Stramonium. So, I really thank you for that case, which was just marvelous. It woke me up to a new realm for Stramonium.

Robinson: *Thank you, Ahmed. I will never forget when you first told me that story. We were sitting in a restaurant in Dallas, Texas. I could have repeated it word for word. That is how deep an impression it made on me.*

Bob Ullman: *What led me to suggest Stramonium for this case was that this woman was not just afraid of death but of the unconscious aspects of death. We can see this in her fear of lakes and pools, which are metaphors for the unconscious.*

Robinson: *Yes. I didn't go into that.*

Bob Ullman: *In addition, I have a story of a "raising the dead" experience, so to speak. My mother died last summer of lung cancer, and I was able to attend her in her final days. She had trouble breathing. Carbo vegetabilis would ease her breathing. We were able to keep her off morphine so that she didn't have to be drugged and she could be as aware as possible. In her last hours she slipped into a stuporous comatose state. At one point, I gave her a dose of what I thought was Opium 200c. It actually turned out to be Opium 10M. It was dark.*

My mother opened her eyes, got out of bed, went to the bathroom, looked me in the eyes, and I think we said goodbye at that point. She got back into bed, closed her eyes, went into a coma, and died that night very peacefully. It was so startling, because she had been completely unable to get out of bed. The Opium appeared to revive her vital force and yet allowed her to die peacefully. It was a very moving experience.

One last comment. I really felt, as people were standing up and giving metaphysical explanations for how Cannabis might be transmitted to the child, that we all know that Cannabis can be transmitted to the child. We know it from our experience. We know it from our souls, so to speak, that these phenomena occur. I think we have to stop apologizing to the scientific community for what we know to be true, for what we know from our experience. Perhaps the mechanisms for all these phenomena have not been elucidated. Nevertheless, we have to stop apologizing for the fact that we do something other than "physical" medicine.

Robinson: *I think it has come full circle. This exchange has shown that we are all, in one way or another, on the way to becoming shamans. I feel this will become more and more obvious as the years pass toward 2000. I have been very moved by your expressions and your sharing. Thank you very much.*

Nancy Herrick, PA-C

A
HOMEOPATHIC
SOJOURN
IN INDIA

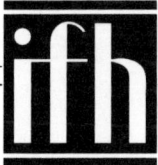

Nancy Herrick earned her master's degree from Wayne State University and her PA degree from the University of California at Davis. She is a co-founder of the Hahnemann Medical Clinic and the Hahnemann College of Homeopathy. Nancy has been practicing homeopathy for almost 20 years, taught for the IFH, lectured throughout Europe, and recently studied with Rajan Sankaran in India.

Animal, Vegetable, or Mineral:
We Are the Remedy We Need

It is always a great honor to come here. This is my favorite conference, because it is an opportunity for all of us to share. No one particularly holds the spotlight at this conference, which is something I really like.

I also want to take a moment to welcome all the European homeopaths who have traveled so far to be here. I want to tell you how much we enjoy having your company, and, please, continue to come. We feel very honored to have you here with us.

I also want to thank Rajan Sankaran publicly for the wonderful work he is doing and the way he has infused the practice of homeopathy with creative ideas that make our work so much more exciting and pleasurable. My experience in Bombay was extremely fruitful. I sat by Rajan's side for four weeks. It was an incredible experience in many ways. I learned different materia medica and about his ways of using potencies, but, most of all, I learned something that is precious, delightful, and yet shockingly obvious. What I learned is that all of life is connected on all levels. And this includes our homeopathic remedies!

Each of us is a living, walking, breathing expression of the remedy we need. We are shouting it from the rooftops through our speech; our handwriting; our clothes; our work; our hobbies; our choices of food, movies, and literature; our parents; our children. I will even postulate that we could find the simillimum from the study of an individual's voice and speech patterns, the whorls on the fingertips, the iris, the tongue, the urine, the stool, the blood. Each part of us contains the whole, and the whole contains each part.

When we perceive what is going on in the patient, then the healing process occurs. We use the mechanism of giving a remedy. That is our tool, but the interaction between the prescriber and the patient has so much to do with what happens in the healing process.

As Karl Robinson has suggested, we are shamans. Traditionally, the idea of the shaman is of someone who has to suffer tremendously, physically and mentally, before he or she can heal others. Well, our suffering has been the years and years of struggling, learning materia medica and struggling with the patients. However, Rajan showed me that the struggle doesn't have to be so intense, that there is more possibility for play, enjoyment, and relaxation in our everyday actions. By sitting there and learning to understand the patient, we can come up with the right remedy.

Of course, we still have to know materia medica and understand the remedies. But if we let go of the tension, of that tightness about getting the right remedy, then we can simply be with the person on a deep level and perceive them.

The one way that I always tended to do work with patients in the past was to ask a lot of questions and to probe, probe, probe. Probing has become less important for me now, less important than listening, observing, and just asking the little questions at the right times. "Tell me more." "What is the feeling behind that?" "What is going on?"

With children's cases, in particular, it is more an expression of fun. What does the child relate to on the deepest level? What resonates for that child? Most children can't relate to the traditional questions. They can relate to what they enjoy, and on that level you can find the remedy.

The remedy doesn't cure us because it's made from pure gold or whale sperm! It cures us because we are a reflection in some very deep way of the essence of that substance and its remedy kingdom: animal, vegetable, or mineral. Lachesis people have a snake-like quality in the core of their nature; Natrum carbonicum people have a mineral-like quality.

If we understand that core, and trust that it is there, we will be much more likely to see it. After I learned this truth, I was shocked at the perfectly obvious signs of my own remedy kingdom that I had never noticed before. I already knew that I was from the plant kingdom because those are the remedies that have worked for me, but when I looked around my living room and saw flowered rugs, chintz chairs, tendrils carved in the wood furniture, roses in the pictures, and dried flowers on the tabletops I began to see the obvious. And they say a homeopath is a good observer!

Ironically, my husband Roger who isn't all that much into decorating has made one strong addition to our decor—his beloved mineral collection. Yes. His remedy is a mineral. These simple tools can help us in that eternal struggle to find the simillimum.

Unfortunately, we are not yet at the stage where we understand any of this in depth. We do not understand how to analyze the whole picture from any part. But what we can do, and what I learned in India, is to use every tool available to us in the beginning of the case to observe the patient and to determine the miasm or kingdom. Then we can spend the rest of the time zeroing in on the simillimum.

By now many of you have heard Rajan speak or have read his books, so you are probably familiar with the idea of central delusion and the use of dreams. What I wish to focus on now is his categorizing of people into animal, vegetable, and mineral kingdoms. He also uses other categories—nosodes, sarcodes, and imponderabilia—but we will not have time to discuss any of these today. I will give you a "word-salad" multi-image list for each of the three kingdoms. This is the way a patient will give it to you in the office.

Most of these ideas come from Rajan, but I have also added a few from my own experience. Remember, these are just ideas, images, and words to help you get a feeling for the type of remedy that may be needed. It's just a guide, not something that is fixed.

Generally, plants don't have structured places where they can go; therefore they are "wandering." They are sensitive and vulnerable to the environment. A plant can stay in the sun or the shade only. If you change its location and it is the wrong location, it will die, even in one day.

The person who needs a plant remedy will tend to adjust to you in the room. If you are getting a little irritable, distracted, or bored, the plant person will notice and will change the topic to something else. If you can tune into that dynamic in your patient, then you can tune into the kingdom.

Most drug remedies are derived from plants. Becoming aware of the characteristics of this category has been particularly helpful for me.

There are exceptions to all of this, of course. Some remedies don't seem to fit well in their particular category. Everyone brings these exceptions up. Just give it some thought. It is, I believe, a remarkable insight. Other homeopaths have had similar ideas, but Rajan has delineated them more fully. It is a very exciting tool that you can use to broaden your scope of understanding.

Animal Kingdom: Attraction and Competition

"It's a dog-eat-dog world."	Malicious
"A bird in the hand is worth two in the bush."	Reactive
	Jealous
Competition	Isolation
Sex	Silk
Connection	Performers
Friend or foe	Advertising
Suspicion	Preachers
To stand out	Lawyers (trial)
To be different	Animal designs
Intensity	Wool
Autoimmune diseases	Fur
Excited	Meat
Kill or be killed	Gulping
Attractiveness	Fish
"I don't understand human beings."	Dramatic
Alert	All or nothing

Snake (Subcategory of Animal)

Throat problems	Water
Suspicious	Kundalini
Clairvoyant	Spirituality
Vivid	Rhythm
Gestures with hands	Oscillation
Problems with teeth	"He speaks with a forked tongue."
Most evolved of animals	"She jumped out of her skin."
Suffocation	

Vegetable Kingdom: Sensitivity and Reactivity

Wandering	Shock
Sensitive	Strain
Gullible	Healers
Malleable	Artists

Vegetable Kingdom: Sensitivity and Reactivity, cont'd

Irritable
"I am sensitive to..."
Adjusting
Flowery
Artistic
Unsteady
Random
Aware

Therapists
Teachers
Quick reaction
Leaves
Cotton
Linen
Nibblers
Blends

Drug (Subcategory of Vegetable)

Tranquil
Benevolent
Praying
Sleepy
Bliss
Industrious-neglect
Hasty-wandering
Courageous-heedless
Analgesia
Exaggeration
Superlatives
Visions
Witty

Poetry
Intoxication
Vivacious
Painful-painless
Beautiful
Confusion
Merging
Nirvana
Colors
Floating
Procrastination
Theorizing

Mineral Kingdom

"We need to get this straight."
Structure
Order
Computers
Not excitable
Family
Business
Bank
Logic
"Hard as a rock."
Hierarchy

Salt
Earth
Slow onset
Steady
Savings
One mode
Home
Something lost
Something failed
Uniform
Business suit and tie

Mineral Kingdom, cont'd

Long time to cry

Organized

Percentages

Chronic complaints

Checks and stripes

Strong feelings easy to pin down

Marriage

Science

Research

Proven

Tried and true

Metal (Subcategory of Mineral)

Armor

"I will battle this illness."

Kings and queens

Crowns and scepters

Gilt-edged swords

Pageantry

War

"It's a fight to the finish."

Weight-lifting

Will of iron

"I will steel myself."

"He seems tough but he has a
heart of gold."

Tanks, planes, battleships

Guns

Mighty

Noble

[Editors' Note: Ms. Herrick's spontaneous explanatory comments, made while presenting the cases, are italicized and bracketed.]

Case Number 1:
A Case Treated by Dr. Jayesh Shah

Female
Age 69

Initial Visit

Chief Complaint: Offensive odors from all discharges (2).

The odors are unbearable for her family (3). Her pathology isolates her from her family.

She changes her underwear four times a day.

The odor is rotten and strong (3). It becomes better for a brief time after she receives antibiotic treatments for her recurrent urinary tract infections (with burning urination).

Her abdomen bloats; she has a sudden and severe urge to pass a stool; she has an explosion of gas, like a bombardment; and then she releases a few drops of liquid stool.

Medical History:
- Worms during pregnancy.
- Breast cancer; operated on; better now. (Note: extreme pathology.)

Her sister died young of breast cancer.

She is highly educated.

Her husband, brother, and daughter are cancer surgeons.

Observation: She sits in a special way and speaks in a very dignified manner as if she were from a royal family.

Industrious. Engages in "purposeful" activity.

She is a Sidi woman (Pakistani) and works in an office with all Marastan men (Bombayettes). There is tremendous conflict between them. "I'm not going to give up to any injustice. I will fight."

Constant fear of colleagues in the office.

She is a no-nonsense person, very firm, disciplined, prompt, dignified. She is never rude or contemptuous. (These are mineral qualities, but the theme of fighting is a metal quality.)

She identifies with girls who have been neglected. She has adopted eight girls.

Fears persecution (2).

When she feels "put down" she has a sense of hammering going on inside of her. Feels her brother is persecuting her. "He put me down." (She says all of this spontaneously.) Her organs feel pounded. "I have had severe sufferings." Hard feelings.

Dr. Shah asks her, "Is it important for you to fight and not give in?" She says, "Yes." Then he says, "Imagine that you don't fight but do give in." She says, "I'm pounding" (3). They treat me like dust" (3). "How can they run over me like this" (2)?

[*"I'm pounding" means that her whole body is pounding just with the idea. As I was explaining the case to Rajan, I made a fist to imitate the patient. Rajan, who did not know what remedy was given, commented, "I'm sure the remedy is a metal if the patient makes the gesture of a fist."*]

To find out the real feeling—the exact dimension—she was asked about her dreams.

First dream: Sees herself as a Kashmiri girl in costumes. Her father takes her for a walk in the jungle, and they gather precious seeds. Her father is a very noble gentleman. ("Noble" and "precious" are words used to describe a noble metal.)

Second dream: There is a huge bungalow on a hill. The sea is all around and it is rising toward the bungalow. People are all around. She tells a servant to bring food and feed them. The water is rising even more. "I try to escape with the jewels, but the valuables are kept with other things. I realize that I should keep my valuables in a proper place." (Jewels and feeding people are images of nobility.)

Third dream: She sees Guru Sai Baba and a beautiful lake with golden lamps all around. She has a nice feeling. The guru comes to her home. (Again, this is a noble image. It is a sign of great significance when a guru wishes to come to your home.)

[*Someone said that you get what you expect. Since I have been home from India, I hear 50 percent more dreams from my patients than before I left. Does this mean all my new patients are now dreamers? No. It means I have an expectation that I will hear dreams. Before, I would have said that most of my patients didn't tell me their dreams or they couldn't remember their dreams.*

Now I expect and pursue the dreams. I will go into even one little dream that they can remember. It is amazing how dreams will open up to you.

Especially pursue dreams with children patients, who are beautiful with their dreams. But they almost always say that they can't remember any dreams when you first ask them.

Don't ask the patient about dreams in a routine way. Wait until they are talking about some deep issue, some emotional point in the case, and then ask. They are much more likely to bring forth the dream when they are in this deep state.]

As a child she was shy, sensitive, and pampered. She held great importance with family and friends; received much love and attention.

Desires radishes and salad (2).

Analysis of Case Number 1

Two themes emerge: (1) performance and nobility, and (2) attack and defense (a strong indication of a metal remedy).

This woman feels royal. She is faced with ego struggle and feels persecuted. She can't understand how others can treat her "like dust." Her body pounds, and then she fights. She is dignified but does not have a big ego. All this indicates a strong metallic quality. It is one-sided. She feels that she can take it all and fight. Her offensive odor and the bloating, gas, and strange stools are so peculiar and such a contrast to her dignified state.

At this point Dr. Shah looked in Phatak under GENERALS, Offensive. There he saw an unusual remedy—Osmium metallicum. Then he looked in Kent's repertory under RECTUM, Flatus, urging for stool, but only flatus is passed. There he saw Osmium metallicum listed as a "1." So he opened the periodic table, and he saw Osmium metallicum next to Iridium, Platinum, and Aurum. He realized that Osmium is a metal remedy and that it is near the precious metals, so the themes of metal, battle, and royalty fit the remedy picture.

Finally, Dr. Shah looked up Osmium in the materiae medicae and found that it fit the case very well:

Phatak: "Secretions are foul."

Clarke: "Urine...like violets.... Sweat...like garlic.... Urging of stool but passes only flatus."

(All the books talk of eructations that smell of radishes, and she says she craves radishes!)

Plan: Osmium metallicum 200c, single dose.

Follow-Up on Case Number 1

All the smells disappeared with one dose and never returned.

She is much better on the emotional level.

The gas and liquid stools also have improved.

Months later she got another bladder infection and that too was cured with a second dose of Osmium 200c.

Case Number 2:
A Case Treated by Dr. Divya Chhabra

Male
Age 28

Initial Visit

(The patient's brother comes in with him.)

He sits still (2), blank (1), and cold (1).

Answers specific questions only.

Doesn't laugh or smile. No expression.

Has urticaria. He scratches it violently until it bleeds.

The itch is violent (2).

Gets severe headaches (2). Heavy pressure on his head (1).

He is tense, but he can't talk about it.

Gets angry often.

He works far away in the deep jungle in the middle of nowhere, building tunnels and tracks for trains. No civilization.

He stays for months without seeing his family. He has no friends. "I work and I sleep. That is all that I do."

He works continuously for two or three days without sleep.

He thinks only of work (1).

He supervises a large crew of men. "If another man doesn't work, my face gets red, I tremble, and I beat him to death. I have to be pulled away."

Observation: He says all this without expression.

"As if it's not in my consciousness." (His brother says that the patient has killed three men. He pays off the police.)

"I lose control" (2). "I feel nothing" (2).

No one talks to him. Everyone is afraid of him.

His brother says that when they were children the patient put a hot iron on the brother's stomach for no reason. No emotion.

"I dislike coming to town." Comes to town only for business. Never asks about anyone.

According to his brother the condition has been getting worse in the last five to six years.

He used to love clothes, shoes, and television.

His brother says that in the past the patient would laugh very loudly and all would laugh with him (2). Now he never laughs.

For the past six years he has had no interest in clothes. Looks scruffy.

His anger comes out at night. "I lose control at night."

If he comes to his home town he does not visit his family. He goes to a hotel, orders beer, and sits for four hours.

[*In Bombay, families are very close. It is unheard of not to visit your family, not to be with your family, and not to call your family all the time. Most families live together. This behavior is striking. He sits in a bar and drinks alcohol. He doesn't talk and just stares at the wall.*]

He has no thoughts at all. Not lonely at all.

Fears snakes (2). "They are not to be trusted" (1).

Won't tell anything to anybody. Can't trust anybody. "Don't know what he or she will do to you."

Fears driving. "I will lose control and have an accident."

Analysis of Case Number 2

The patient displays the following traits:

- Violence in all his expressions.
- Totally isolated; mistrusts all people.
- Sneaky.
- Detached.
- Feels all people are his enemies. All are out to attack him. When touched, he feels like someone hit him.

This is beyond metal and beyond most animals. This behavior is so extreme that it fits only the limited picture of a spider. The extreme isolation and violence and the lack of any emotion about these characteristics is very spider-like. His only fear is of snakes because they can't be trusted. This distrust is a definite animal clue; survival of the fittest. Snakes come out during the day, and spiders come out at night. Spiders don't have friends. If you put two spiders in a box together they will fight to the death. Spiders catch and kill even when they aren't hungry. Baby black widows are left with nothing to eat but each other and out of 100 maybe 25 will survive.

He is hard, cold, and isolated. He kills to survive. He lives in a jungle, in a tunnel. Scorpions are just like this. They are totally detached. They only work. Scorpions are enemies, not to be trusted. They are still, cold, hard, and then they sting. They can go for days without food or water. They come out in the night.

The proving of Scorpion done by Jeremy Sherr showed a fear of accidents when driving, an ability to concentrate on only one thing at a time, and a tendency to be accident prone. A Scorpion person is totally detached and disconnected from the human race. The world is a picture. They share a different view and don't want to join.

Other Scorpion traits (from the proving) are as follows:

- COLD, HARD, PIERCING EYES, staring.

- Mind concentrates on one object only.

- Tunnel vision.

- Feels separate.

- Out of control.

- Terror, panic, fear.

- Surge of violent emotions at trifles.

- Impulses to hurt others.

- Everyone is a creep.

- Dreams: Hostile to those around him. Stinging comments. Someone trying to murder him, and he sank needle to bone. No remorse. Heads chopped off.

- Killing without remorse. More than a snake.

- Everybody is an enemy.

- If you leave a snake alone, they won't trouble you. But a scorpion sees all as the enemy and will attack.

- Torture if stung. Horrible pain from the sting.

Plan: Scorpion 30c, single dose.

Follow-Up on Case Number 2

He wept for ten minutes (2).

Feels terrible about not caring about anyone. Feels very emotional and upset.

[*Divya, the prescriber, was afraid that the patient was suicidal because he was so upset about the life he had been leading. But, of course, to feel this way is the only possible human reaction if he is to come back to health. If he felt happy at this point, something wouldn't be right.*]

His face looks less angry, much softer and more expressive.

No violence.

He talks to people and smiles now.

He visited his family for two weeks. He bought new clothes for the visit.

His headaches are somewhat better.

He had been diagnosed with tuberculosis in the past. When he was four years old he was treated by allopaths for it. Now his troubled breathing is back.

[*This case provides an extreme example of a patient who needed an animal remedy and who responded quite dramatically. The patient was essentially brought back into his humanity.*]

Case Number 3:
A Case Treated by Dr. Rajan Sankaran

Now, let's look at a different type of case. I saw Rajan take this case in January of this year (1994). The patient has had very good results from the remedy, although the follow-up interval is now only six months. [Editors' Note: The patient continues to do well as we go to press, 12 months after the initial visit.] I want to share this particular case with you because it is an excellent example of the thinking process Rajan and his colleagues use.

Male
Age 38

Initial Visit

He is a policeman.

He has suffered from right-sided trigeminal neuralgia for the past ten years.

It began a year after a motor accident (2). He sustained blunt injuries when a bus overturned.

Observation: He is wearing stripes. He has red eyes and long incisors. Looks like a boar.

Desires sweets (3).

Saliva drools from his mouth.

He snores in his sleep.

Afraid of dogs.

Observation: Shows a slight grimace around his mouth.

His mouth, especially the angle of the mouth, is worse from touch (2), from drafts (2), and from eating.

He takes one to three pain pills daily.

Otherwise, he is healthy.

He wants to avoid surgery (1).

Dreams of hitting someone, burning someone. "Someone is hitting and burning. They call me. I catch them, and I hit them. I feel very bad about this, very stressed out, but this is my work. I have to do this. I am a policeman.

[*Initially he says there are no dreams, but he remembers once Rajan pursues it.*]

He is easily and suddenly affected by an accident (3). If he hears a scream from inside his house (2), he rushes inside with the feeling that someone is on fire, someone is dying, someone is suffering. A tremendous tension.

When someone screams, he feels shocked in the chest (2). "I always overreact."

When guests are visiting in his house he's constantly afraid that their little children will fall over the railing.

He has been afraid of jumping from railway platforms for the past two years (1). Afraid of falling (2).

He will not let a small child run free because he is afraid that a car will run over the child (1). "If I leave him, something will happen." So he holds the child's hand.

Afraid of accidents (3).

He's constantly afraid while on duty that if he has to leave for some reason, another officer will check that he's not there. "I must go back to my duty." If he is late for work, he is anxious that he will be reprimanded (1).

If he hits or slaps a criminal during the course of duty, he repents the rest of the day (2). "Why in anger did I do this?"

If he shouts while at home, he thinks about it the rest of the day and wonders why he did that.

When he eats, the first morsels are painful; as he continues to eat, the pain gets much better (1). But if he starts to eat again ten minutes later, it's painful again.

He wants to be totally alone when he eats (1). His family is a nuisance; they disturb his eating, which is already painful.

He can't enjoy food because of the pain; can't eat freely.

He salivates in his sleep.

His condition is worse from shouting and screaming (2). He wants silence (2). (Sensitive.)

Sleeps well.

"I want quiet" (3). He is worse after a quarrel or fight (3).

He tells his wife not to shout because he's afraid the neighbors will hear. "Our respect will be lost."

He is asked why he's a policeman. [*This is the first direct question in the interview. Rajan asks, "Why are you a policeman? It seems like the wrong job for you."*] "I hate it (3). My father wanted me to be a policeman. I was put there, but I have to leave it."

He can't tolerate the other policemen. Doesn't like their manners (1). They are dishonest and harass others.

He has so much sympathy (2). He lets offenders go. "I catch them and don't lock them up."

He would prefer to have his own business. "I tell people to never get into this profession—ever!"

If he catches people breaking the law and they ask him for forgiveness, he will let them go. But if they're belligerent and tell him not to touch them or say that they know someone in the government and that the patient will lose his job, then he will surely take them to the police station.

He hates bribes (3). He is mostly honest and upstanding.

He doesn't smoke; doesn't chew betel nut or tobacco. People respect him and he likes it (2).

"I don't like what other policemen do. They force people to give them bribes." I accept what I get (1). I don't put pressure on people for bribes. I believe such money turns into sickness or loss. I never steal, yet I have this illness. It's because I take money dishonestly. If I take money, I fall sick (2). (Superstitious.)

His relatives respect him. He doesn't do anything wrong. "I feel satisfied that I have the respect of all. I don't feel like doing dishonest things. My wife respects me. No alcohol or womanizing."

When the pain gets too severe he feels suicidal (1).

"Why is this illness after me when I have not harmed anyone" (3)?

He is against the police department. "If anyone asks, I would expose them. I hate this department."

The public reputation of policemen is bad "whether you do good or bad." He is stamped as dishonest and drunk just because he is a policeman. He is very troubled by this (3).

His eyes are always red from the pollution (3).

"I hope you're not reporters and are going to tell the newspapers." (He asked this at the end.)

[*Yet, he told the whole story before it occurred to him that I might be a reporter.*]

"No holidays. Policemen are the busiest. We can take off only on days that the children are in school and it's raining. No freedom (3). They will call me to duty any time."

Perspires a lot (2).

Analysis of Case Number 3

At this point in the case, Rajan said, "I have not even a faint idea of what the remedy is, but I will work it out." This in itself was very interesting, because in most of the cases that I observed he felt very clear about the remedy after taking the case. What follows is the thought process he went through in arriving at the prescription.

His predominant traits are as follows:

- Moral.
- Superstitious.
- Wants respect.
- Punished by guilt.
- Desires peace.
- Sympathetic.
- Sensitive.
- Fears accidents.
- Anticipation as if something bad will happen.

There is tension on the nerves, and this creates the trigeminal neuralgia. If anything touches him or moves near him, it causes immediate pain (1). He is very sensitive (3). It seems clear that he needs a plant remedy, for the following reasons:

- Sensitivity is the first feature, not structure.
- His problems lie along many axes. There is not just one theme or idea.
- He doesn't display the attraction and competition features of the animal group.

- His talk is unstructured.
- Sudden pain and sudden symptoms. (Usually a plant characteristic.)

[*I read you the whole case because I wanted you to note how he changed subjects constantly. He talked about his pain, about his family, about his job, about his children, about his sensitivity, and about his guilt. Many themes came up randomly throughout the case. The talk was very unstructured. He rambled through the story of his life. This suggests a plant remedy.*]

So, he needs a plant remedy. But what kind of plant? He has a fixed job and a fixed neuralgia. He has an issue of secretiveness and guilt, hiding behind an image. This all suggests the sycotic miasm.

We must therefore look for a sycotic plant remedy. Staphysagria comes to mind first. It is sycotic. Rajan felt that Staphysagria would partially help in this case, but it does not have the suddenness of this patient's state. We need to look for something that has a sensitivity to sudden noises.

Rajan looked up sensitivity to sudden noise in the *Synthetic Repertory*, and only Borax was listed. He did not think this was a Borax case. He said, "We need to find a remedy that is both a sycotic plant and very sensitive to noise. The starting from sudden noise and the intense shocked feeling in the chest express his general state, and the remedy must have this."

He looked at the rubric, MIND, Starting, noise, from. Nux vomica is there (bold type). Staphysagria is not listed for this symptom. Both Nux and Staphysagria have sensitivity to insult. Nux vomica is a remedy that is both a plant and sycotic. It has the patient's sensitivity to sudden noise as a marked element in its picture. Staphysagria may fit the overall picture better, but Nux vomica has many aspects of the patient's characteristic state:

- Worse from drafts and touch.
- Wants to be quiet.
- Desires composure and tranquillity.
- Gets angry when interrupted.
- Cannot bear noise.
- Trembles with anger (Both Nux vomica and Staphysagria).
- Desires to strike.
- Worse from contraction.
- Suicidal tendencies.
- No courage.

If a bigger man approaches him, he strikes out first and then repents later. He does not suppress his feelings. He always lets them out. The big difference between Nux vomica and Staphysagria in this case is that this man does not suppress his feelings. It all comes out, which is the opposite of Staphysagria's characteristic state. Staphysagria holds in. This man told his whole story and then worried about me being a reporter!

The tension on the nerves—with the shock sensation in the chest—the need for respect, the violent tendencies yet expressing regret, and the oversensitivity to draft and to noise indicate a plant and the sycotic miasm. It all adds up to Nux vomica. This was Rajan's reasoning.

Plan: Nux vomica 1M, single dose.

Follow-Up on Case Number 3

Since the Nux vomica, the trigeminal neuralgia is dramatically better. It is essentially gone at this point.

I especially wanted to present this case because it gives us a feeling for how we can, step by step, work through the analysis of the remedy. This is quite a difficult case. Many of us would have given Staphysagria, yet Nux vomica is the remedy that acted.

Mary Caselli: I am a bit confused. Animals are fighters, too. How do you tell the difference between an animal and a metal remedy in terms of the fighting?

Herrick: With metals, it is a general theme of battle. With animals, I think it is more the idea of competition. It is a one-to-one fight, an attraction and competition, and a desire to win in this private combat. With metals, it is a larger issue of overall battle with the world, not the feeling of attractiveness or of showing off.

Jennifer Jacobs: When you are talking to children about their dreams, do you have the parents in the room? And at what age do you not have the parents there?

Herrick: At first, I usually interview the parents with the child to get some general impressions, and then I try to spend time with the parents alone and with the child alone. Under about age six, I let the child tell everything with the parents in the room. Over age six, I usually like to have it more private.

Also, children will often tell you a bit more when they are alone with you.

Laurie Dack: *I want to ask you about the first case. I don't understand how the one symptom that Jayesh used to direct him initially, that he looked up in the repertory, was representative of the themes that you were describing.*

Herrick: *His explanation was that the idea of the offensiveness was so striking for someone who saw herself as royal. It made the offensiveness so painful for her.*

Laurie Dack: *The offensiveness as a general symptom, that I understood. I was asking about the specific symptom of the flatus. How is that representative of the case?*

Herrick: *That was, I believe, a simple matter of looking up a specific symptom, part of her chief complaint. In other words, he was merely looking under her symptoms to see if there was any unusual remedy there or any remedy that struck him. This is something we all do frequently, but he was immediately tuned into that remedy because of his way of thinking.*

Laurie Dack: *I was wondering if we could in any way understand that symptom in the context of how we perceive the case.*

Herrick: *In terms of a metal, you mean?*

Laurie Dack: *I mean in terms of a metal or in terms of this particular woman and the juxtaposition between the nobility and the offensiveness.*

Herrick: *Well, what do you think?*

Laurie Dack: *I don't know. Did he make any comments about this?*

Herrick: *No. He didn't make any specific comments about it. It was just that for someone with a sense of nobility it would be particularly difficult to be offensive, so this was a very striking symptom. It was almost a kind of "karmic" symptom, perhaps, that she would have this particular aspect. That was the most difficult thing for her to have, given her state. It could be seen as a polarity. The polarity idea is very important in case analysis.*

Karl Robinson: *The Scorpion case was fantastic. It is, however, tempting to think of a "cold-blooded" metal like Mercurius for the case, because of the* *nighttime aggravation. Mercurius is also known to kill. And there is the syphilitic component, the antisocial component of Syphilinum. Scorpion was obviously the best remedy, but I don't know how I could arrive at the prescription.*

Herrick: *One thing that strikes me about the case is that the man would strangle with his bare hands. There was no knife. There was no metal brought into it. If he stabbed, then we would have to think more about a metal. He strangled with his bare hands, just like an animal uses whatever it has as a part of its body.*

Barbara Newlon: *This woman who prescribed the Scorpion must have been familiar with the remedy. I was wondering how she would have known, because Jeremy Sherr just proved this remedy one or two years ago.*

Herrick: *No. I think it was longer ago than that.*

Audience: *Eight years.*

Barbara Newlon: *There was some confusion over on this side of the room. People were looking for Scorpion in the materia medica and couldn't find it.*

Herrick: *The Complete Repertory has many additions for Scorpion. But, yes, this is a problem. Obviously, many of us will be doing provings on new remedies. Disseminating the information will continue to be a problem. I assume there will be further additions to the Complete Repertory and other computer programs as time goes on. In this way, we can keep building our knowledge. It is one of the great advantages of the computer world.*

Barbara Newlon: *I think it is so important that more provings be done, because then we notice people who require those remedies. It is so necessary.*

Herrick: *Yes. The people who need these remedies are out there. We need to do more provings, and we need to understand these remedies much more deeply. We will also find that, as animals become extinct, it becomes more important to do provings on them. We need to understand these animals. Rajan made a very interesting point. He believes that as an animal becomes extinct, its energy, which must remain on the earth, will go into humans. This energy has to be manifested, so humans will "become" these creatures. Actually, he feels that this is true for anything that becomes extinct, plants as well.*

Anne Schadde: *I can imagine how it was for you in India, because I spent several weeks there studying with Rajan some years ago.*

I want to share a very small case I observed in India on the third day after I arrived. We were sitting in his school, and a man came in to be treated. He was a very simple man who complained of a sore pain in his chest that was worse from touch.

He spoke in Hindi. Rajan got this one symptom and translated it to me. After one minute, he asked, "And what is your profession?" The man responded, "I push a wheelbarrow." He carried things around for others. Rajan then said, "Fine, thank you." He was finished with the case taking. I said, "How can you take a case like this?"

Rajan said, "Give it to the students." His students then got more information from the man, which they related afterwards. This man had only one son, who had married some years ago. Marriage is very important in India. Suddenly, the young wife died after only half a year of marriage. But they had spent all their money to celebrate the wedding. No money was left. The woman is very important in India for preparing and serving meals, and for so many things. After he heard of his daughter-in-law's death the man developed this severe pain. He couldn't work anymore and they didn't have any money. This is a very difficult kind of situation in India.

Rajan said, "The first rubric I took was ailments from pecuniary loss" (from the Synthetic Repertory; *the remedies listed include Arnica). The man expressed his state through his symptom—a sore pain that is worse from touch. This is an Arnica symptom. He even had an Arnica job, pushing a wheelbarrow all day long and straining his muscles. The remedy was Arnica, a very "simple" prescription. He gave him Arnica 10M. Two weeks later, I saw this patient again. He was smiling. He could work. He was fine. For me, the case was a miracle.*

Herrick: *Yes. It is a way of thinking that is simple yet very deep. It pervades the case. It is beautiful, and it has really strongly affected my prescribing. I hope in a year or two I will be able to bring you many of my own cases that elucidate this way of thinking.*

One other thing I didn't emphasize is the idea of talking to patients about what they enjoy, what is fun for them, what they are deeply involved in. This is another marvelous way to penetrate the case. I had a case of a little girl whose favorite activity was looking at her posters of fish. She said, "Every night before I go to bed, I look at my fish posters. I read about a different fish and I stare at it right before I go to sleep." I knew that her mother's remedy was Sepia. Based on these aspects, I gave the girl Sepia with beautiful curative results. We are an expression of our remedy.

Ahmed Currim: *I think the master (Hahnemann) indicated some of what you are describing in article three (of the* **Organon***). "If the physician clearly perceives what is to be cured in diseases, that is to say, in every individual case of disease, if he clearly perceives what is curative in medicine..." It is all there in article three. It is not a new idea, but it is a new way of looking at it.*

Herrick: *Yes. Clear perception. Thank you.*

Roger Morrison, MD

THREE PALLADIUM CASES: EXPLORING THE ESSENTIAL ELEMENTS

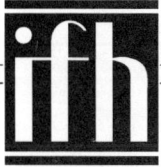

Roger Morrison studied homeopathy extensively with George Vithoulkas in Greece from 1982 to 1984. He is co-founder of the Hahnemann Medical Clinic and the Hahnemann College of Homeopathy. Roger is a popular lecturer in Europe and North America, and a respected author of homeopathic materials. His most recent book is the popular Desktop Guide to Keynotes and Confirmatory Symptoms.

Introduction

We are going to talk about Palladium today. I will be presenting a video case in a moment. But, first, let's look at two paper cases.

[Editors' Note: Dr. Morrison's spontaneous comments, made during his case presentations, are bracketed and italicized.]

Case Number 1

Female
Age 38

Initial Visit

At age 28, she was diagnosed with pituitary adenoma that was causing acromegaly. It was diagnosed because of the growth of her jaw. She had surgery, which made her much worse. The surgery disturbed her adrenal function, and she had to take cortisol for some time.

She had a pelvic and abdominal growth, which was surgically removed. It was a right-sided, grapefruit-sized growth thought to be endometriosis. It was visible to the eye.

She currently has a tender left ovary (3). Worse from steps.

[We have many clues suggesting Palladium. First, a right abdominal growth. A right ovarian cyst, growth, or tumor is a big hint for Palladium. Also, after the growth was suppressed, it went to the left ovary. This is very common. You can take an ovarian cyst off one side, but it will come back on the other side. For ovarian cysts that are tremendously painful from jarring, the first remedy we think of, naturally, is Belladonna. When it is not Belladonna we think of

Palladium. Another minor point is that Palladium has delusions of being enlarged, so there may be some connection with the enlarged jaw.]

Her menses are heavy with some clots. They last three days and are getting worse. She has been getting a second period at mid-cycle for the past three months.

She has PMS. It was worse when she had a stressful job. Since she was laid off she feels better. She becomes sensitive (3), easily offended (3), and irritated (3). She would get angry at work, but when the same situation arose outside of the PMS time it would not bother her. She also has tension, fullness of the abdomen, and fatigue before her period.

[*She attributes her sensitivity and irritability to the fact that she is premenstrual. The rest of the time she is "fine." So many times you will hear this. I used to ignore these symptoms, thinking that because they occur just before the period they don't count. But when you really delve into the matter, whatever is wrong before the period often turns out to be the main problem. This is when the pathology comes furthest forward. So, please do not ignore the "premenstrual" symptoms.*]

Has had two dramatic episodes of fatigue with daily napping. Worse from exertion or unusual activity.

Knee pain (2) and elbow pain (2).

Becomes depressed when the weather is cloudy. Better from the sun.

Worries about practical matters.

[*Here is a hint for a mineral remedy. She is oriented toward the practical.*]

"Intelligent, articulate, aware."

Focuses on her goals and then achieves them.

Sees all sides of an issue.

Wants to have it all—children, job, domesticity.

She is very sensitive. Takes offense easily (3). Gets "put out or bristly."

"Outspoken, direct, blunt, pointed."

She never means to hurt others. Assumes she's being criticized (often incorrectly) and retaliates.

Organized and clear.

Appreciates people and life.

Happy.

In her present job she's uncomfortable and nervous because she thinks that she can't do it.

Feels she keeps herself from succeeding (although she talked her way into the position).

Ambitious about home and family.

She never thought she would have to work.

[*What does that sound like? Royalty—just as in Sankaran's description of patients needing a metal (mineral) remedy.*]

Would like to be single and live alone.

Afraid of burglars in the past.

Craves potatoes (3), pasta (3), and bread (3).

Plan: Palladium 1M, single dose.

Follow-Up

The problems with fatigue, the irritability, and the other emotional dysfunctions resolved.

The ovarian problems also resolved.

The Subtle Arrogance of Palladium

A description of the demeanor of this first Palladium patient is instructive. She came in and was extremely cheerful and bright, almost professionally bright. She kept up this cheerful demeanor all through the interview. Even when she was talking about serious problems, she was smiling frequently and trying to stay very upbeat.

The real story with her job stress is that she constantly felt that people were insulting her and not appreciating her. She had the feeling that she should have been promoted. She also had the feeling that people did not say "hello" warmly enough when they walked by.

This is a very strong characteristic of Palladium. Why are they so cheerful? It is because they expect the same from other people. If a Palladium says, "Hello, I am so happy to see you this morning," and you walk by and just grumble in your usual morning fog, this is taken as a deadly insult. They feel tremendously insulted that you didn't greet them in a bright, shiny manner.

This is part of the subtle arrogance and haughtiness of the remedy. It is not the haughtiness of Platinum. It is not that type of more overt egotism. The subtlety is in their expectations. They take offense at the least thing. If somebody criticizes their work in any way or if they even think that someone has criticized their work, it is a great insult. "Ambitious" is another good word to describe Palladium.

Case Number 2

This case was taken by Peggy Chipkin at the Hahnemann Clinic. It shows a slightly more extreme side of Palladium.

Female
Age 73

Initial Visit

Chief Complaint: Severe depression.

Her problems began after a family dispute in which she had a huge fight with her son over his treatment of his son, her grandchild. She felt he was not sufficiently affectionate toward her grandson. Her son screamed at her and she yelled back. "I cried, I got angry, and I went off my rocker. I couldn't believe what I was thinking. If I had had a gun at that moment.... It just seemed like the only solution. I wanted to kill him and then kill myself."

[*She weeps, sighs, and sobs occasionally as she tells all of this.*]

"Now I don't feel like doing anything. I feel terrible inside. I haven't done the cleaning for two weeks. I don't want to get out of bed. I sit and watch soap operas."

Her husband reports, "She is depressed and angry, worse and worse over the past several years. Homeopathy is like a religion to her."

[*I have seen this several times in Palladium patients. Homeopathy is indeed like a religion, in a particular way. For example, you prescribe a remedy and the patient comes back on follow-up and tells you that the remedy helped a lot. However, when you inquire as to what specifically is better you find that the complaints are actually not better. The patient reports improvement because they want you to like them. One of the most important issues with Palladium is that they want approval from others.*

So, in this way, homeopathy can become a religion for them. It doesn't matter whether they get better from the remedy. The main thing is that they have made contact with you. They want you to feel that they have been a good patient, that you approve of them, and that they have made you happy. All of this enters into their thinking.]

The husband continues. "She is not the same person she used to be. I try to please her, but she accuses me of doing the opposite of what I know she likes."

[*The poor husband! He gets up in the morning. He tries to get her the breakfast she wants. He brings it to her. "Why do you bring me this in my room? You think I am not capable of getting up on my own?" Whatever he does, she feels insulted.*]

The husband says she is very critical. "She can scream so loud it scares me. Yet, she was able to be her usual self when a niece came and visited for a few days."

[*The niece stayed with them for several days. The whole time that she was there the patient was able to act perfectly cheerful. She got up in the morning and didn't watch soap operas all day. After the niece left she collapsed into bed, totally depressed. When she goes out to dinner with friends she seems to feel fine, and then she comes home and has go to bed.*]

She is irritated if anything goes wrong.

She is offended easily.

She has a history of ovarian tumors and fibroids.

Plan: Palladium 200c, single dose. Later, another single dose of Palladium 1M was required.

Follow-Up

After Palladium this woman experienced a dramatic resolution of her symptoms. She began to function normally, and the whole situation with her son was resolved. They reconciled.

This kind of response is common with this remedy. After Palladium is given, the patient often resolves a dispute. He or she realizes that the argument was over practically nothing and that there was no real substance to the argument. It was only a disagreement of perception.

Palladium: The Core Elements

I want to give some of my impressions of this remedy. I will also add in well-known information.

Palladium is a rare metal. It is chemically related to platinum. When it was first discovered, in fact, the early chemists and alchemists were not sure whether it was a separate substance from platinum. They thought it might be the same substance in a slightly different form.

Because it is a metal, it will have the characteristics of metal remedies that Nancy (Herrick) mentioned earlier in her presentation. One Palladium patient of Nancy's had a repeated dream. The essence of the dream was the image of a sword. The sword was inlaid with many beautiful patterns in pure gold, with an ornately carved handle. It was the sword of a king or a royal person.

It is a metal sword. This makes us think of a metal remedy and of the theme of battle. I think you can clearly see the theme of battle in the two cases we have looked at thus far. The first woman was having battles at work. She would get offended and insulted.

The second woman had a long drawn-out fight with her son and also battled with her husband.

The main theme in Palladium, of course, is the *feeling of being insulted or neglected*, of not being considered "enough" by other people. Palladium, as I mentioned earlier, is found with platinum in nature. Platinum is the "beautiful sister" of Palladium, the one that gets all the attention. Palladium is the one that gets ignored. It is not as beautiful. Is that going too far? No, everyone seems ready for this kind of artistic speculation (audience laughter)! It is interesting, at any rate, that both Platinum and Palladium are used primarily with women patients.

The main state can be described with the following images: imagines herself neglected; feels slighted in any circumstance; pride is easily wounded. Another rubric that comes up is "desires flattery." Flattery will definitely get you somewhere with Palladium. It will get you exactly what you want.

The good opinion of other people is so important to Palladium. (In the repertory it is under the rubric, Longing for the good opinion of others). When you spend so much time and energy trying to get the good opinion of other people, you can easily feel humiliated or mortified. (Palladium is in bold type for ailments from mortification.) You can feel neglected and discontented.

The second theme is excitement in company. They have to put on an image. Image is everything with Palladium. If they go out to a party or are in a social setting, they act happy and cheerful. In Boericke, it is described in this way: "Keeps up brightly when in company, much exhausted afterwards, and pains aggravated." This describes it exactly. Remember Case Number 2. The woman was severely depressed but kept up a good appearance the whole time that her niece was there. The outside world was there in her house. She put on an act of being happy, but as soon as the niece went home she collapsed into her true depressed state. For Palladium, problems come on from the effort of keeping up a good appearance.

In Case Number 2, we also can see to what extreme the anger will go. Palladium is known, of course, for irritation and anger, but Palladium can also take the anger to the point of rage. They have many complaints from becoming angry. They may use violent language, have violent imagery. This woman wanted to shoot her son. Again, the metal imagery comes through. She wanted to shoot the son and then shoot herself, which reminds us of another metal remedy, Aurum metallicum.

There is a strong tendency for weeping in Palladium.

Underneath, there is a feeling that they have to perform. This is another character-istic of a metal remedy. They must perform well or other people won't like them. This is how it seems to them.

"Obstinate, tries to appear amiable." This rubric from the Complete Repertory captures the whole flavor of the remedy. This is very characteristic. They may give you a cheery "Hi, how are you doing?" but underneath there is a strong will and a desire to get their own way. The woman in Case Number 1 is ambitious. She is "ambitious about home and family." She wants things done her way, yet her very pleasant manner and appearance do not reveal this. The smile is nearly glued in place.

Here is a sample dialogue:

"No, I am sorry, Mrs. Smith, we cannot find an appointment for you. You will have to wait until next week."

"Oh, but I really wanted an appointment this week."

"I just don't have anything in my books."

"But, you know, Dr. Morrison, I just really feel I need an appointment this week!"

"Well, okay, Mrs. Smith, let's see if we can find one in here somewhere."

Physical Characteristics of Palladium

There are not many strong physical confirmatory symptoms for Palladium. The most common are the ovarian cysts, especially right-sided ovarian cysts, but it can easily be ovarian tumors.

The connection with the pelvic area is so common that you have to wonder a bit about prescribing Palladium if you don't see some sort of urogenital problem. It may be endometriosis. It may be ovarian neuralgia without actual ovarian enlargement. The pains in the ovary are worse from jarring, worse after the menstrual period, and worse from or after excitement. They are better from lying on the back and bending the legs back, and sometimes better from lying on the left side.

We can see many other pains in the same area, such as in the uterus. The patient may describe the pains as knife-like or cutting. Again, this suggests the imagery of a metal remedy. The pain is better after a stool. Other symptoms are strong dysmenorrhea, uterine prolapse, and heaviness in the pelvis (such as we see with Sepia), with a sense of uterine prolapse. They also may have shooting pains from the navel to the pelvic region, better from pressure, and bladder pains, worse from exertion.

Palladium also has a characteristic headache. The headache is like a band. It is different from other remedies with band headaches, which are horizontal around the front and back. The headache of Palladium goes vertically over the top of the head, like a band going from ear to ear or from temple to temple.

Audience: Where is that symptom found in the repertory?

Morrison: I don't know. It is in the materiae medicae, but I don't know where you find it in the repertory. [Editors' Note: One place in Kent's repertory is HEAD, Pain, vertex, extending, ear, from one to other.]

Remedy Differential

Let's briefly discuss the other remedies you are likely to confuse with Palladium.

Pulsatilla

Believe it or not, and this is very telling, the first remedy you are going to confuse with Palladium is Pulsatilla. It is the remedy most commonly misprescribed for Palladium. Why? Because Pulsatilla needs approval and tries to win you over. They need your affection.

With Pulsatilla, it is a forsaken feeling. With Palladium, it is a neglected feeling. This is a bit "less" than forsaken. There is a slight but very important difference. In clinical practice, feeling forsaken versus feeling neglected often doesn't seem that different. However, there is a significant distinction to be made.

Forsaken means that inside the person feels a loss, that they don't have your help when they need it. Palladium feels that they don't have your respect when they demand it. You see the difference? Palladium shows a certain "smallness" of mind. The things that Palladium "needs" are not the things that we would ordinarily consider very important, such as requiring a proper smile in the morning in order for our friendship to continue.

Palladium can carry a long-term grudge. They have a big fight with somebody. Later, the other person tries to reconcile and the Palladium person will outwardly comply. But they don't forgive inside. This is similar to Nitric Acid, not forgiving.

Why don't they forgive? It is because the person didn't apologize. It has to be in this way, "Please accept my most humble apology." If the person doesn't come forward with this exact format, it is completely negated by Palladium. It doesn't matter that the person's whole spirit was one of reconciliation.

On the other hand, if someone comes up and says, "I owe you an apology for this," Palladium is satisfied even though the apology was not given in the true spirit of reconciliation. Because the "apology" was made, the Palladium person is satisfied. The concerns of Palladium are the concerns of someone who is more concerned with image than with reality.

Both Palladium and Pulsatilla are remedies that weep a lot. Palladium will frequently weep during the interview. Both remedies have many difficulties with the female tract. It is very easy in practice to confuse these two remedies. In Palladium, there is a greater hardness and resolve, a stronger will than we characteristically see with Pulsatilla.

Apis

The next remedy you will mistake for Palladium is Apis. Why? Because the physical symptoms center on the right ovary—pain, swelling, and so on. Any problem with the right ovary can be Apis or Belladonna. Like Palladium, Apis is an extremely irritable and strong-willed patient, easily offended.

In addition, there is a common element of jealousy. I am treading on thin ice here. You will not find Palladium listed for jealousy, even in the magnificent Complete Repertory. Still, you can see that the whole spirit of Palladium is such that the patient could be extremely jealous. If they see that someone is paying more attention to another person, they will be jealous. We will see this in the video case that I will show you in a moment. But Apis has a different sort of jealousy. [Editors' Note: See Dr. Morrison's discussion of Apis in the 1991 IFH case conference proceedings.]

If you just look at the symptoms superficially—jealousy, right ovary, irritable, easily offended, and menstrual problems in a strong-willed type of person—you might give Apis instead of Palladium.

Platina

Of course, Palladium can be confused with other metal remedies. I pointed out some similarity with Aurum metallicum. There are great similarities with Platina, but there are also great differences between Platina and Palladium. Platina does not need other people's approval to the same extent. This is because they already know that they are superior to you! Why should they care if you approve of them or not? Platina does not usually struggle for other's good opinion in the way that Palladium does.

Though both remedies can have female problems, particularly ovarian problems, Palladium is not typically an oversexed remedy and Platina is.

The desire for flattery is present in Platina, but they will take it as their due in the natural course of things. Palladium feels the need for the flattery, because it is "under" Platinum.

Phosphorus

Another remedy you can confuse with Palladium is Phosphorus. Can you imagine that? On the surface, both are bright and cheerful. Palladium patients are so engaged with you from the moment they walk into the office. Yet, there is an element of manipulation because they want your good opinion and approval. Phosphorus people are engaging just because it is their nature.

Phosphorus can also have a lot of trouble with the ovaries and the female tract.

Feeling easily insulted is not a strong feature of Phosphorus, although Phosphorus can feel as though love is not returned to them.

Belladonna and Lycopodium

Two other remedies one might confuse with Palladium are Belladonna, as I mentioned earlier, and Lycopodium, because of the right-sidedness and the haughtiness.

Case Number 3

Female
Age 42

Initial Visit

She has had asthma for the past five years.

She had been living in a damp bedroom and cold house (3).

She has two teenage daughters. She had been raising them as a single mother and was under a lot of stress. Many arguments. She has felt better since one of her daughters moved in with her brother-in-law.

Yelling at her daughter caused her to lose her voice (3).

There was much turmoil and anger over her daughter's disobedience, especially over staying out late. One day she walked into her daughter's room when she was gone. The daughter had not left a note. The room was a terrible mess. The idea came that perhaps the daughter was involved with drugs, so she started to search the room. Just then, the daughter returned and found her searching. A big fight ensued, and the patient began wheezing for the first time. She has never been completely well since this time.

At that moment the patient felt that she got "no respect, no consideration, and no communication."

"The way she would leave her room and then take off...and then I would see her, and I interpreted no respect for me. The least she could do is keep her room decent. But, I guess when you stop and think about it, if I look for something then I am going to find something (to be upset about).... I just sort of felt...she just didn't care. There was no respect, no consideration. There was little or no communication, and I am very sensitive."

She also gets asthma attacks when she fights with her boyfriend.

Worse from excitement (2), anxiety (2), and hurrying (2).

"I am tough in a way, but then I have my periods where I am very weak and very sensitive. Sometimes people see the toughness, and they don't realize that I am very sensitive underneath. When they shoot things at me it affects me. I am trying to work on it, to realize that it is outside of me, but it is hard when you get close to someone and they do that."

[*This describes the Palladium state very well. Remember Case Number 1, where the woman had very strong opinions and described herself as outspoken yet was also very sensitive and easily offended underneath? This is what this patient is saying. People can get at her very easily. She can be made to feel bad about herself easily.*]

She has a stressful work environment. Feels mental abuse (3), humiliation (3), and rejection (2). Feels left out (2).

[Editors' Note: The following is an excerpt from the video that Dr. Morrison showed during his presentation of this case.]

> **Patient:** This is the type of person that she is (co-worker). But when I realized that it was just aimed at me and nobody else was getting the same kind of treatment, I finally spoke up to management. She seems to realize that this is how she can get at me.
>
> **Morrison:** By saying nasty things?
>
> **Patient:** Yes. She is rude and abrupt. It is a three-girl office, and it is not a very professional atmosphere. When management comes to visit, everybody is "Ms. Nice Person." When they come and go, it is just like night and day.
>
> **Morrison:** Are you on equal levels at the office, or do you work underneath this other person?
>
> **Patient:** I work underneath. It is an odd situation. When I hired on, she wasn't hired as my supervisor. She was just another person there, and the job description was that I was going to have my own accounts and my own responsibilities. I was just going to work with this other woman. Well, you know, it was different when I got on the job and she had total control. She wasn't training me.
>
> **Morrison:** What sort of work do you do?

Patient: Clerical—shipping, receiving, data input work.

Morrison: So, she didn't train you?

Patient: She didn't train me at all, except for what she wanted me to be totally dependent on her for, and I played her little game.

[*So, she is hired at the same time as another woman. The other woman wanted to take all the control, and the patient says, "I played her little game." This is part of the mentality, playing little games. Oscar Wilde once said that the politics in a small college are so vicious because the stakes are so small. This describes the state of mind.*]

Patient: Eventually, I thought she would let me be on my own. Well, it never came about. In the meantime, we got computer work and computers and yet she was doing all the training and she was just letting me do certain parts of the work. I thought we both were going to get equal training. It didn't work out that way.

[*She didn't get training equal to the other woman in doing this "important" task of logging in the entries of the orders that came in. You see, she was slighted. That is what she is saying. "She got more than me. She got to train with the computer, and I didn't get to train with it." This is the feeling.*]

Patient: I talked to our boss one time, and he finally clarified the situation. He just said at that point, "Well, she is not your boss." But that was not the impression he had led me to believe and it wasn't the way that they had been working it for the last three years. So, that was kind of stressful for me because I wanted to have my own responsibilities, to get a little recognition. I can't seem to please her.

[*"I can't seem to please her." This is the feeling. They need the other person's approval. And they need recognition. It comes up again. It is just written all over every one of her interactions—with her children, in her work. It doesn't matter. Whatever the interaction is, these same feelings will be there.*]

Patient: We have a problem communicating. I like things being told simple and straightforward. She goes "around about" in a lot of ways. Basically, I figure maybe she has an analytical mind or she is projecting problems that are not there. It has nothing to do with what she is trying to have me do at that point, and I have to try to keep bringing her back.

What I feel is that I will give her words to explain something, and she will use my words, but they are like simplified words or simplified meanings. I say, "You mean this, this, and this?" and she says, "Yes, I mean that, that, and that."

Morrison: She mimics you, in other words?

Patient: Right, and I got to the point that I didn't ask her anything anymore after a while, because I just didn't want to go through that demeaning type of training.

Morrison: And it triggered an asthma attack because you felt...

Patient: Exasperated and stupid. I wondered why something like that would occur and with me only?

[*The other woman is apparently trying to clarify what she said, and the patient thinks that she is mocking her. She feels insulted when insult is not intended. In the repertory, feeling stupid is "mortification." She felt mortified, and then came the asthma.*]

Morrison: What about the other woman in the office?

Patient: She seems to communicate with her just fine. I listen to the way she talks to the other girl, and she talks to her in a completely different way than how she talks to me. I tell myself that I'll be quiet and I will be a "yes" person. Maybe that will help, but it doesn't. I don't worry about it. It is just that I feel bad because I am there eight hours a day. The two are buddy-buddy, and I am the third person, right?

[*"I am the third person." The same feeling keeps coming up. You can't make her into anything else other than Palladium.*]

Patient: If I want to get into a conversation I have to make the effort to do it, but she talks directly to this other person. So, at times, I feel left out and I feel kind of bad and rejected and all of that. But, I think that I am an adult and this is the way it is. I can't let it affect me, and it doesn't affect me too much. I get upset only when she starts criticizing my work and starts training me as if I am a child and talking to me on that level. Then I turn off, and then I am seething. And, before I know it, I have my asthma.

[If you look in your repertory under the rubric, Asthma, emotions, from excitement, you will find Palladium, along with a few other remedies.]

> **Jonathan Shore:** *What's striking is that this rubric is the only place where Palladium appears in the entire RESPIRATION section of the repertory. It is the only respiratory symptom for Palladium in Kent's repertory and in the Complete Repertory.*

Her asthma also gets worse from cold, damp weather (2) and smoke-filled rooms (2).

Gets hot and perspires during the attack (2). Feels she can't get air (2). Wheezes (2), but no coughing.

High cholesterol (288).

Good energy.

Warm-blooded.

Gets hot flashes (2), especially in the morning.

No thirst (2).

Craves lamb (2), fish (2), salty food (2), salted lemons (2), sour food (2), and spicy food (2).

Averse to fat.

Eating shellfish causes her to break out in hives (2).

She sleeps well. On her back (2). Stays covered.

She never remembers her dreams.

She kicked her husband out because of his alcoholism.

Independent.

She had a hysterectomy in 1978 because of a cyst on the uterus or perhaps on the right ovary. Before then, her menses were okay.

Her sex drive is okay. She has more interest than her boyfriend.

Afraid of rodents.

She is organized (2), irritable (2), impulsive (2), and happy.

Past history of seizures at age eight or nine. They would come when she was angry or when crying for sympathy.

Plan: Palladium 200c, single dose.

Follow-Up

Three months after the remedy was given, she was using her inhaler two to three times per month instead of two to three times per day at the time of the initial interview. She had experienced a significant improvement, which continued.

By the one-year follow-up, she had completely stopped using her inhalers.

I have been treating her now for about three years. She comes in once a year and has continued to do well. She has had one more dose of Palladium 200c in the time I have been seeing her.

This case clearly demonstrates the main elements of Palladium. It is not a huge remedy, but it is one that can easily sneak by you if you don't know what you are looking for. The physical pathology in this case is typical of Palladium, in that the asthma was not horrible. It was significant, but not horrible. The physical pathology is rarely terribly advanced with Palladium cases.

> *Barbara Newlon: I had a case of a small child. She was two or three years old. Both parents came in with the child. My initial impression was that she must be Phosphorus because she was so bright and happy. It was so interesting to me that you mentioned Phosphorus in your differential. I don't remember the particulars. I think she was brought to me for chronic ear problems and frequent colds.*
>
> *One thing that struck me during the whole interview was that it was nearly impossible to get information from the parents because this child demanded so much attention from them. As soon as I started to ask them questions this child*

realized that she was not getting any attention and she would demand the attention in some form. It was intense. There were not many modalities or particulars that would point to Phosphorus or Pulsatilla or other likely remedies. I gave Palladium, and the result was a good cure.

Morrison: *The specific physical pathology doesn't matter that much. This is not what you are going to base your prescription on.*

Sheryl Kipnis: *It occurs to me that perhaps Palladium is a remedy for the victim that one doesn't feel sorry for.*

Morrison: *Absolutely. I think that describes it perfectly. You can feel a certain type of sympathy, but even as they are telling the story you feel there is another side to this story.*

Judyth Reichenberg-Ullman: *I think what you are saying about subtlety is important. I finally discovered one of my patients needed Palladium. I had given her Lycopodium and Apis without result. She had right ovarian complaints, but I never thought of Palladium. I had thought Palladium was so much like Platina that I totally missed it. Then, when I listened to her very carefully, her slighted feeling came through. It was nothing that jumped out.*

Morrison: *That is exactly my experience, although it can be more pronounced in some cases. Generally, Sulphur will be one "octave" below the haughtiness of Platina, and Palladium will be another "octave" below Sulphur. It is more tempered and less apparent than Platina in most circumstances. Sometimes the haughtiness will be quite prominent. Sometimes you will hardly notice it.*

Palladium's haughtiness is mostly seen in what they expect of others rather than in the way they act toward you. You rarely get the feeling that the Palladium patient feels superior to you. The haughtiness is in the constant need to be included, the constant need to be flattered or paid attention to. In this sense, it is a passive sort of arrogance rather than the aggressive, negative arrogance that we usually associate with Platina.

Audience: *Have you seen any cases of males needing Palladium?*

Morrison: *I haven't prescribed it for a man yet. I think it must also be needed in men's cases, although much less frequently.*

Valerie Ohanian, AHCH

TWO CASES OF OBSESSIVE-COMPULSIVE DISORDER

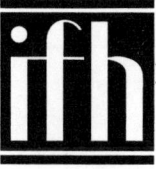

Valerie Ohanian has been practicing classical homeopathy for 12 years in Minneapolis, Minnesota. She completed the IFH Professional Course in 1985 and graduated from the Hahnemann College of Homeopathy in 1989.

Seeing Through the Obsession to the Simillimum

Obsessive-compulsive disorder is certainly not a new phenomenon. Early homeopaths documented its symptomatology in the provings and in the clinical literature of remedies that correspond to the syphilitic miasm.

In the last few years, I and many of my colleagues have seen more and more of these kinds of cases, with increased severity of symptoms, and I think that homeopaths will have to deal with even more of them in the next decade. Why the increase? It is hard to pinpoint a single cause. A history of childhood sexual or physical abuse is part of many of these cases. Extreme self-esteem issues are central to others. A fear of loss of control escalates to pathology in yet others. The rise of syphilis in our culture also may be a contributing factor.

This condition is generally considered to be the result of great violation—massive invasion of personal boundaries at a young age. Even though symptoms don't necessarily appear in childhood, the disorder is in place. A great stress will often bring out the condition later in life.

Regardless of the cause, most of these cases are not simple cases of excessive hand washing. Competent clinicians, both allopaths and homeopaths, find them difficult to manage and cure. However, we can cure them with homeopathy once we see through the obsession to the simillimum.

These patients present elaborate defense systems, so elaborate that it can be difficult to find your way through the maze of symptoms. Finding the thread that leads to the underlying disturbance can seem nearly impossible, but it is my experience that once the thread is found and the disturbance understood, these cases actually progress quite rapidly to a cure.

It takes a great deal of acceptance and lack of judgment on the part of the homeopath to elicit symptoms in these cases, especially to get to the nuances of feeling and thought. People with these disorders often have a lot of shame about their inner worlds, and they will censor themselves if they detect the slightest hint of discomfort on the part of the practitioner. They may come back for a few visits, but the practitioner will never get the full story. So, be especially careful.

I will present two cases. Both cases are significant, because they involve very deep, long-standing pathology that was quickly cured with a single remedy and they add to our knowledge of the curative remedies.

Case Number 1

Female
Age 50

This is a very, very pleasant woman who lives in an upper middle class suburb. She has successfully raised four children and works as a legal secretary. She and her husband divorced amicably ten years ago.

She has been struggling with her symptoms for six years. During that time she has sought treatment by psychotherapists, nutritionists, and psychiatrists, who helped her to manage to some degree. Her most recent treatment was electroshock therapy, which didn't do anything but "wipe out" her short-term memory. She says she is quite depressed because of her symptoms.

The initial interview was conducted in two sessions. She was, repeatedly, very afraid that she had said something inappropriate or horribly offensive. Each time this happened it took a great deal of time to reassure her and get her back on track.

First Interview

She is feeling very depressed (3).

"It's hard to cope. My inner reserve is empty."

Gets hot and sweaty if she thinks she has made a mistake (3).

She was so discouraged last week that she cried and cried. "It was such a relief to get it out, and that someone was with me."

She will cry easily if she has someone to talk to who understands her.

Has a heavy feeling (2) in her arms and legs.

Starts to perspire when she feels panicky or afraid (2).

Her sleep is poor; wakes between 1 and 3 a.m., even when she takes sleeping pills; takes sleeping pills often.

Her sadness is worse in the morning.

She has a compulsive need to do things over and over—to fix them.

"I sometimes feel everything I do is wrong. I harangue and criticize myself (3) all day long. I'm constantly shaming myself."

Feels heaviness (3) in her chest when she criticizes herself.

"I fear something bad will happen. I fear making a mistake. I fear expression. I fear intimacy."

She had a bad review at work. "It was shattering to come up with a bad review. I feel the need to prove myself all the time at work since I got the review. My self-confidence is zilch. This review really set me back, but my boss tells me not to worry about it."

She is not focused. Couldn't concentrate (3) after her hand accidently brushed her supervisor's shirt. Obsessed that she shouldn't have done that.

Afraid that she doesn't say goodbye and hello in the right way to people (3).

Rips up checks because she doesn't think she has signed them properly.

Feels guilty all the time (3).

"I don't ever feel that I'm really good at anything."

Afraid of touching people (3) because something bad might rub off on them.

She is overly aware of cleanliness (3). Washes her hands all the time (3).

"I'm not working things out inside myself."

She needs to be perfect. If she walks on wood chips instead of the walkway she feels she has done something very wrong and can't shake the feeling for days. Yet, she has some impulse to walk on the wood chips. "I need to be perfect, and I need to be bad."

"I've been reading a lot of books, like *Compassion and Self Hate* by Dr. Rubin, and I've decided that I am scrupulous, unsure, hesitant, rigid, and legalistic."

She felt terrible yesterday because she drove around a 10-mph curve at 15 mph. She goes over this in her mind again and again; wants to do it over and fix it.

"I feel that I'm lower than everyone. I'm tired of feeling so needy and helpless."

Takes an anti-inflammatory drug for an aching pain in her right hip. Starts to perspire if she thinks that she has taken the drug five minutes later than the prescribed time, because she feels she has done it wrong.

Feels guilty (3) if she inadvertently hears conversations of others. Feels bad for eavesdropping.

Afraid she will infect others with her "germs" (3). Afraid of contaminating things around her (3). "If there is a possibility that my underwear could have touched a chair I was sitting on, I know I've contaminated it and I feel horribly ashamed. If I breathe on a paper and then someone else touches it I feel horrible. I can't stop thinking about it for days."

She also obsesses about the remote possibility that she might have done something wrong. "What if I breathed on somebody? What if I missed seeing a stop sign?"

Second Interview

Her appetite is poor. No particular food cravings, but she does like to eat ice cream at night.

She has a history of poor digestion, and has been treated by a chiropractor for it over the years. Occasional nausea (1), gas and bloating (2), and cramping and diarrhea after eating (2). Was told it was candida.

She went through menopause four years ago. No associated symptoms. Not using hormones.

For several years she has experienced heaviness in her chest with heart palpitations at night (2).

Her physical energy is good.

She was feeling a lot of grief (3) around the time the obsessive-compulsive disorder started. Worked as a medical receptionist then and realized that she had "deep, deep feelings" for a regular patient there, a very wealthy, influential married man. She kept these feelings to herself because "it would have been wrong to have a relationship and, besides, it was impossible." Her manager noticed the friendship she had with this man, however, and criticized and teased her about it one day in front of the entire staff. "Since then, I started tumbling down. I quit that job, and things have been horrible since. I'm so sick and tired of it. I've tried everything."

Analysis of Case Number 1

This case was troubling to me. The pathology was severe. This woman couldn't even breathe without having terrible feelings of remorse and self-hatred. The electroshock treatments had failed. The next likely course of allopathic action would be confinement to a psychiatric ward. So, I felt more than the usual need to be correct in my remedy selection. And, yet, the case didn't seem clear at this point.

So far, I thought the appropriate rubrics were as follows:

- MIND, Anxiety of consciousness.
- MIND, Remorse.
- MIND, Reproaches, ailments after.
- MIND, Reproaches, himself.
- MIND, Grief, ailments from.
- CHEST, Palpitation, heart, night.
- CHEST, Oppression, night.
- RECTUM, Diarrhea, eating, after.
- ABDOMEN, Pain, cramping, eating, after.

These rubrics yielded unsatisfactory results. I used MacRepertory, both including and excluding polycrests. Including polycrests yielded Pulsatilla and Aurum metallicum as the top remedies (Figure 1). Eliminating polycrests brought up Aurum metallicum followed distantly by Aurum arsenicum (Figure 2).

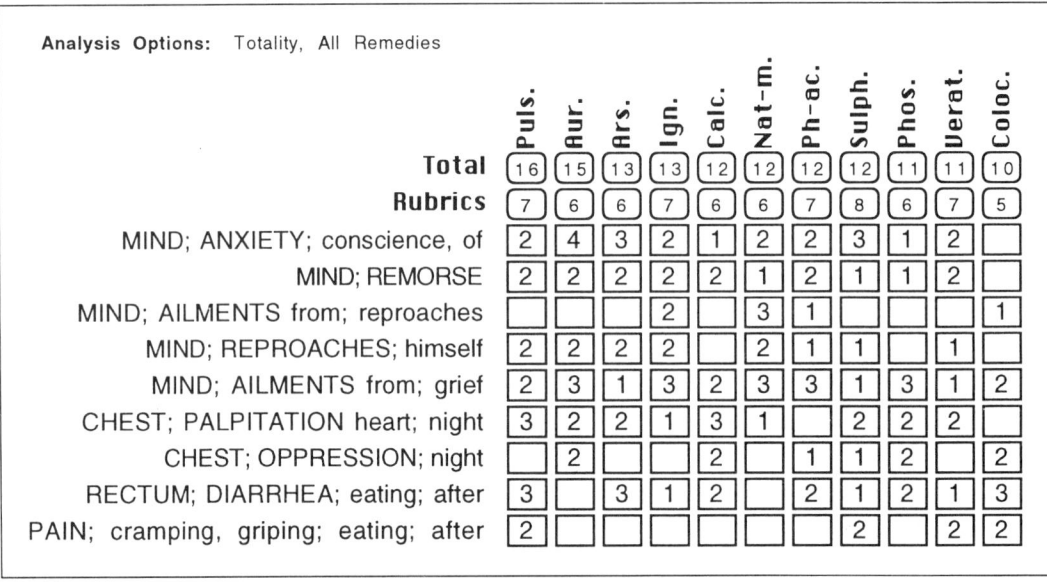

Analysis Options: Totality, All Remedies

	Puls.	Aur.	Ars.	Ign.	Calc.	Nat-m.	Ph-ac.	Sulph.	Phos.	Verat.	Coloc.
Total	16	15	13	13	12	12	12	12	11	11	10
Rubrics	7	6	6	7	6	6	7	8	6	7	5
MIND; ANXIETY; conscience, of	2	4	3	2	1	2	2	3	1	2	
MIND; REMORSE	2	2	2	2	2	1	2	1	1	2	
MIND; AILMENTS from; reproaches				2		3	1				1
MIND; REPROACHES; himself	2	2	2	2		2	1	1		1	
MIND; AILMENTS from; grief	2	3	1	3	2	3	3	1	3	1	2
CHEST; PALPITATION heart; night	3	2	2	1	3	1		2	2	2	
CHEST; OPPRESSION; night		2			2		1	1	2		2
RECTUM; DIARRHEA; eating; after	3		3	1	2		2	1	2	1	3
PAIN; cramping, griping; eating; after	2							2		2	2

Figure 1

Analysis Options: Totality, 25 polycrests

	Aur.	Ign.	Ph-ac.	Verat.	Coloc.	Op.	Dig.	Staph.	Alum.	Cocc.	Hyos.
Total	15	13	12	11	10	10	9	9	8	8	8
Rubrics	6	7	7	7	5	4	5	5	5	4	4
MIND; ANXIETY; conscience, of	4	2	2	2			3	1	3	2	2
MIND; REMORSE	2	2	2	2			2		1	2	2
MIND; AILMENTS from; reproaches		2	1		1	4		2			
MIND; REPROACHES; himself	2	2	1	1		2	2				2
MIND; AILMENTS from; grief	3	3	3	1	2	2	1	3		3	2
CHEST; PALPITATION heart; night	2	1		2			1		1		
CHEST; OPPRESSION; night	2		1		2	2			2		
RECTUM; DIARRHEA; eating; after		1	2	1	3				2	1	
PAIN; cramping, griping; eating; after				2	2				1		1

Figure 2

At this point in the case I thought the remedy was an Aurum salt, probably Aurum muriaticum or Aurum muriaticum natronatum, because of the intensity of the grief reaction at the onset of her symptoms, but I wasn't sure yet. So, I asked the patient the following questions:

- Have you made any serious suicide attempts? (If this were an Aurum case, she probably had tried—given the intensity of her symptoms.)

- Have you ever had bleeding uterine fibroid tumors?

- Did you have any grief associated with your divorce, even though it was amicable?

She said that two years ago she had overdosed on sedatives and alcohol. She probably would have died if a friend hadn't found her and called an ambulance. She had withheld this information for fear I'd send her back to her psychiatrist.

In response to the second question, she said that seven or eight years ago, prior to menopause, she had started to have flooding menstrual periods. She consulted a gynecologist, who diagnosed uterine fibroid tumors and prescribed birth control pills. She took them for over a year. The bleeding didn't resume, so she forgot about the problem.

And, finally, she admitted that the breakup with her husband was difficult even though the divorce was "friendly." She felt terrible when her husband told her he wanted a divorce. She had trouble believing it at first. She couldn't understand why. They had a good sexual relationship, and she loved him. After the separation she would think about him and long for the past. This went on for years. It would be especially bad after her children would talk about him.

She finally started feeling a little better. But then her impossible feelings for the patient at work combined with her supervisor's criticism brought on the deep depression and the obsessive-compulsive symptoms.

On the basis of this new information I chose Aurum muriaticum natronatum. Both this remedy and Aurum muriaticum can show suicidal tendencies and severe ailments from romantic loss, but the bleeding uterine fibroids differentiate in favor of Aurum muriaticum natronatum. Other symptoms in this case that help confirm the remedy are the cramping and diarrhea after eating and the sense of oppression in the chest at night.

Plan: Aurum muriaticum natronatum 200c, single dose.

Characteristics of Aurum Muriaticum Natronatum
and Aurum Muriaticum

George Vithoulkas describes the feelings surrounding romantic loss in both Aurum muriaticum natronatum and Aurum muriaticum:

> If there is a breakup in the relationship they stay with intense feelings and longing for what they lost. Eventually they go into depression. They are full of emotion and nostalgia. They can't get their mind away and the depression goes deeper (Celle Seminar, 1991).

Vithoulkas says these remedies don't have the suicidal tendencies of Aurum metallicum. However, this has not been my experience, both in this case and a couple of others. It has also been said that the remedies don't share Aurum metallicum's strong sense of duty and responsibility, but my case certainly illustrates the pathological extremes of responsibility associated with Aurum metallicum.

This case also illustrates Aurum muriaticum natronatum's relationship between emotions and hormonal activity. Vithoulkas says the hormonal system in these patients works full speed, faster than normal. After the sudden stoppage of emotions, as with withdrawal of romantic love, the hormones keep working to the point of producing huge swellings such as uterine fibroid tumors.

Finally, Aurum muriaticum natronatum is considered to be the most sympathetic Aurum. It doesn't have the aggressiveness of the other Aurums. It can be refined, sensitive, perceptive, warm, and communicative. These patients can look like Phosphorus, with their anxiety and desire to establish connection. This was certainly true in this case.

Follow-Up on Case Number 1

Six Weeks After the Remedy

Her position at work was eliminated. "I was sad, but I handled it well."

"I'm basically very sad now. I feel all the sadness of a lifetime. I don't feel suicidal, but I'm asking why I should want to live. I'm questioning my ability to experience love in my life. Part of me wants to live so much. I'm aware of how deep my self-hatred runs."

Her fear of contamination is better, not as powerful.

The heaviness in her chest continues, but the palpitations are less intense and less frequent.

Plan: Wait.

Ten Weeks After the Remedy

"I still feel like I'm improving quite a bit, but I have minor panic attacks if I get a crumb or a grain of salt on a piece of paper."

She has had some heaviness in her chest and a few palpitations the last couple of days, otherwise not noticeable.

She has a new job and is coping fairly well, even though training is not provided.

Vaginal bleeding for the last ten days (an old symptom).

Plan: Wait.

Fourteen Weeks After the Remedy

"I'm really doing better. I'm not feeling overpowered anymore."

The vaginal bleeding has continued, but appears to be lessening.

The perspiring is mostly gone.

No palpitations.

"I have a sense of hope that I'm really moving through this."

Plan: Wait.

Five Months After the Remedy

The vaginal bleeding has stopped in the last month.

Feeling stronger.

Much less afraid of making mistakes, even at work.

Plan: Wait.

Seven Months After the Remedy

Her appetite is very low.

Perspiring a lot; wakes up wet in the morning.

"I know I'm real compulsive. I can look in an envelope three or four or five times to make sure nothing is in it. I mistrust my senses. I'm sick of the pain. I'm very angry I have these symptoms."

Assessment: Even though she is a bit worse, there is no significant relapse.

Plan: Wait.

Eight Months After the Remedy

"I'm incredibly better. I'm doing really well and am incredibly pleased with myself."

Occasionally feels she is contaminating things, but she isn't so ashamed and doesn't get obsessive about it.

Her relationships are really good.

She has close friends now and is considering getting back together with a man she was seeing last year. "I feel I can handle it now."

Plan: Wait.

Twenty Months After the Remedy

Telephone consultation.

She is doing very well. She has a job she likes and is in a relationship.

She feels quite strong and will call if she ever needs to.

Assessment: Needless to say, her response to homeopathic treatment was excellent. She needed only one dose of the remedy in over two years, in spite of her history of birth control pills, antidepressant drugs, antipsychotic drugs, and electroshock therapy. Even though this remedy isn't usually associated with obsessive-compulsive disorder, it appears to be the simillimum in this case and has acted curatively.

Plan: Wait.

> *Judith Coates: Was this woman under any psychiatric treatment at the time that she saw you?*
>
> *Ohanian: No. She had been on four or five antidepressants at various times and had quit them about two months before she came in. That also made me nervous. As you know, when people stop antidepressants on their own they can become precipitously worse.*
>
> *Karl Robinson: I am very interested in this case. I give a lot of Aurum metallicum in my practice, but I don't see Aurum in the way you saw it here. I really can't penetrate into the case the way you did. Could you review your thinking again?*
>
> *Ohanian: Sure. I saw the Aurum thread in the extreme degree of guilt and remorse and in the feeling that she was not achieving. For her, achievement was whether she folded an envelope correctly or typed a letter exactly right. This is not a "big" Aurum symptom, in terms of being in the world. It is much more "small-minded." These elements, combined with the depression that led her to a very serious suicide attempt, turned the balance for me toward the Aurum family.*
>
> *Karl Robinson: Was there any religious component to it?*

Ohanian: Not at the time I saw her. She wasn't despairing of salvation in a religious way, and so on. She did make a couple of off-handed comments about possibly being sexually abused by a minister and being mixed up about God early in life. There may have been an issue about that, even though it wasn't in the front of her mind.

Murray Feldman: I have given Aurum muriaticum successfully in several cases where I have seen a cross between Aurum and Natrum muriaticum characteristics. Recently, I was looking at a case with Lou Klein and he suggested Aurum muriaticum natronatum. The case was a cross between Natrum muriaticum and Aurum. I had to be honest and say that I did not know how to differentiate clearly between Aurum muriaticum and Aurum muriaticum natronatum. I haven't had enough experience with the two remedies. I was wondering if either you or anyone else has been able to differentiate between these two. Why not prescribe Aurum muriaticum in this case?

Ohanian: I can give you a fairly simple answer to that. I gave the Aurum muriaticum natronatum because she had that strong symptom of bleeding fibroid tumors in the past.

Murray Feldman: Yes. When the patient doesn't have the tumors, I have stayed with Aurum muriaticum.

Ohanian: Without that symptom, I would have been hard-pressed to give the remedy, although she did have what I considered to be a Natrum feature. She was closed down emotionally; she had a protected sense about herself. That is also, I think, why I had to have her come in for a second interview. She was reticent to express her feelings. She would talk about her feelings in a fairly clinical way, but the feeling wasn't there.

My colleague Eric Sommermann, who has a PhD in biochemistry, and I have discussed the chemical differences between Aurum muriaticum and Aurum muriaticum natronatum. Eric, would you say a few words about that?

Eric Sommermann: It is a peculiar thing, because Aurum muriaticum, of course, is just the salt. It is simply gold chloride. Aurum muriaticum natronatum is Aurum muriaticum that has been co-precipitated with some Natrum muriaticum (sodium chloride). It appears to be no more than a mixture of two salts that have been co-precipitated. I have not been able to determine if there is a separate crystalline structure for this particular preparation. When salts precipitate, there is sometimes a specific and unique stoichiometric crystalline structure.

I cannot tell if there is a special structure for Aurum muriaticum natronatum. I have not been able to find all the literature on how it is prepared. If there isn't a distinct crystalline structure, then it is one of the rare remedies in our materia medica where we have just mixed two together and called it one remedy.

I have thought a lot about why fibroids are particularly associated with the Aurum muriaticum natronatum. I can't answer that. I wonder if Aurum muriaticum also would cure fibroids. [Editors' Note: Both Aurum muriaticum and Aurum iodatum have been added for uterine fibroids in the Complete Repertory. The source was Boericke's repertory.]

We may be using two remedies when one would work. I know some people have differentiated some fine points between the two remedies, but I am not sure about it. If anyone does have information on how the remedy is made, I would be very interested in learning about it.

Jonathan Shore: *I just remembered a case where I gave Aurum muriaticum natronatum and it seemed to work quite well. However, the patient and I did not get along well at all, and she left me and went to see my wife. My wife couldn't read my writing (audience laughter) and gave her Aurum muriaticum, which also worked very well for her!*

Barbara Newlon: *I had an Aurum muriaticum case. This was a woman in her 60s. She came to see me after having seen a very good homeopath who had given her many remedies. I gave her five or six remedies that did her very little good. She continued to see me. Finally, I sat down with the case and looked at it simply. She had heart palpitations at night and a deep despair that she always talked about. I gave Aurum muriaticum, and she is now doing very well on LM potencies.*

Ahmed Currim: *What connection do you see between Aurum muriaticum natronatum and Syphilinum? I am reminded of a patient who had similar complaints, to whom I gave Syphilinum. She made me change the paper on my examination table twice, once because I put my hands on it after sneezing and once again because she put her feet on it and said she didn't want me to work on her case. I really puzzled over her case, and I finally gave her a dose of Syphilinum because she was always washing her hands. But she never came* back for follow-up. I heard from others who said that she was really much better, but I felt I didn't help her. Now that I hear your case, this patient comes to my mind. If she comes again, and I think she will, then I will see if I can fit this remedy to her. It is just wonderful that you give a case and I remember a patient that I didn't help.

Ohanian: *In this kind of obsessive-compulsive case, we can frequently get caught up in the symptoms. Hand washing can mean a lot of things. The question is, "What does it mean in each individual case?"*

With this woman, she washed her hands not because she was so concerned about cleanliness or her own health but because she was afraid of contaminating others. So, that was important in my understanding of it. I think there probably is a syphilitic component in every obsessive case like this, but you have to differentiate carefully to find the appropriate remedy.

The grief in this case was very important, and that really led me to an Aurum salt. As she herself said, her symptoms started to come on when she had to leave a Natrum muriaticum-type of relationship. It was an intellectual relationship with a male patient where she worked. She knew it was hopeless. She could never have a love relationship with him, and then her boss exposed it. She had to leave her job, she grieved over leaving this patient, and then the symptoms started. When we look back further in the case, we find that she was grief-stricken about the end of her marriage and hadn't really gotten over that.

Guy Kokelenberg: *We had in our working group a case just as you have described. The remedy was not Syphilinum, not Aurum, and not Silica. It was Curare, which has the rubric, Delusion, dirty, everything is, that. The case was cured with Curare. A very strange remedy.*

What has struck me in quite a few Aurum muriaticum cases is that there is a desire for company. This is something we don't usually see with either Aurum metallicum or Natrum muriaticum. The Aurum muriaticum patients are depressed, but they have a desire for company and the depression is ameliorated by company.

Ohanian: *That is my understanding. In this case the woman said the one moment of relief she had in years was when she could cry with a friend.*

Case Number 2

Female
Age 35

In Case Number 1 most of the obsessive-compulsive symptoms were focused inwardly, in a syphilitic type of expression. In Case Number 2 the symptoms are focused outwardly.

I first saw this woman ten years ago. At that time she came to me because she had genital herpes, contracted when she was raped a few years earlier. She also had nightmares of being sexually abused, feelings of suffocation in groups of people, and a frequent sense that someone was behind her, either just following her or ready to attack. Her short-term memory had not been good since the rape, and she had long periods when she couldn't focus. She would have "wild" fantasies about being violent toward men and sexually abusing them. She was given Medorrhinum 200c. The herpes greatly improved, as did her general sense of well-being.

She came back three years ago with more extreme problems. She had done fairly well for a number of years. Then an older woman she was very close to died, and her mind started to unravel.

Initial Visit

"I guess I didn't handle the grief well. I got so angry I felt full of rage a lot. Then I started having problems with my mind."

Problems in perceiving—seeing and hearing. She mistook the size of one fork next to another. People's eyes looked cockeyed.

Wakes suddenly in a hyper-alert, fearful state between 1 and 3 a.m.

Terrifying dreams: brother pours acid on her father's head and the head melts away.

"I'm losing my thoughts and my short-term memory."

She is seeing psychiatrists and has been diagnosed as "psychotic" and "obsessive-compulsive." This is frightening to her, so she decided to try homeopathy again.

Herpes is not a problem.

"I would kill if I were a man. I would rape. I have balanced this desire by being strict with myself and kind to others."

Her body is tense. She jumps if massaged around her hips. Doesn't like to be touched.

"Along with the darkness coming up in me, I'm remembering this evil thing. When I'm about to fall asleep I have hallucinations. Dolls are jumping off the shelf and are coming to kill me. I hear voices in my head just before I fall asleep."

"I'm obsessed with killing and hurting people. I can't get these thoughts out of my head. I have very violent fantasies. A lot of them are about my therapist and about men. I want to kill and hurt them. I bought a gun, and I'm taking a class to learn to shoot it properly."

She can't stop the violent thoughts and she is getting more and more depressed.

"I've started to get obsessed with killing myself, to get away from these fantasies. I really could hurt someone, you know. I'd shoot myself. One bullet to the mouth and one to the temple."

She has been suicidal before, but has never been able to do it. "The main thing in my mind is responsibility. People depend on me. My nieces. You just can't do that to people."

She is more worried about hurting others than hurting herself.

"I've got to this point of losing feeling. I try to keep a conscience, but it's hard. I'm talking in a matter-of-fact way because I'm studying myself."

"I want to shoot people who get promoted at work. I want to go on a warpath and hunt someone down."

She has fantasies of raping people, and the fantasies are very sexually exciting to her. "I'm brutalizing in my fantasies. I get the best orgasms this way. I feel sexual and masturbate, and when I do it turns to violent thoughts. I feel such a weakness inside myself."

She is quite ambivalent about her sexuality. She feels sexual attraction toward men, yet she is in a sexual relationship with a woman.

Has violent dreams—being slashed on the legs, being stabbed in the shoulder to death, being stabbed by voodoo dolls.

Has fits of rage (3); throws her body against door frames. Feels rage only when alone. Has difficulty expressing anger with others.

Painful menstrual periods (2), with hot flashes and feverish feelings. Perspires (1) before menses.

She has migraine headaches during her periods and has trouble focusing (2).

Eats compulsively (3).

Desires bread (3), ice cream (3), cheese (3), and sweets (3).

Picks the skin around her fingernails (2).

> *Ahmed Currim: As I looked at a few rubrics in the repertory, the remedy that came to mind was Platina. I took ailments from anger and silent grief. I thought about the size of the forks not being perceived correctly. I also looked at ailments from grief, desire to kill, suicidal but lacks courage, violence, masturbation, dreams anxious and frightful, aversion to touch in Generalities and touch aggravates. Platina also has waking at 3 a.m.*

> *Guy Kokelenberg: I forgot my repertory, so I feel a bit "naked." I thought the first sentences were very important in what you wrote here: "I guess I didn't handle the grief well. I got so angry I felt full of rage a lot. Then I started having problems with my mind." So that is an etiology for me. Another thing that struck me was, "I feel sexual and masturbate and, when I do, it turns to violent thoughts."*

> *For these reasons and because of the stabbing aspect, I thought of Staphysagria. I have many Staphysagria patients who have fantasies about stabbing. Staphysagria is, of course, a remedy for stabbing wounds, too. Stabbing sometimes has sexual connotations.*

Karl Robinson: *I used these rubrics: Delusion, has to murder someone (a new rubric in Synthesis, in which we find Arsenicum album, Hepar sulphuris, Hyoscyamus, and Lachesis); Fear of killing (Absinthium, Alumen, Ammonium muriaticum, Arsenicum album, China, Derris, Hyoscyamus, Mercurius, Nux vomica, Rhus toxicodendron, Sulphur, Thea); and then Desire to kill— a huge rubric. Did she want to kill with a knife or a gun?*

Ohanian: *A gun, although I think a knife would have done well, too.*

Karl Robinson: *And then I looked under Suicidal and Vision, illusions of vision. By this time, I was thinking of Hyoscyamus. Hyoscyamus is there. It is also under Objects seem too small and Objects seem too large. These symptoms, coupled with rage and the sexual elements, lead me to think perhaps Hyoscyamus would be a good prescription.*

Murray Feldman: *She didn't just want to kill. She wanted to hurt, she wanted to rape, she wanted to violate, and she wanted to mutilate. So, I looked up dreams of mutilation, combined with desire to kill, rage, lasciviousness, and masturbation. All of these lead me to consider Mercurius, which exhibits the horrible violent impulses, the suicidal and homicidal urges, and the syphilitic aspect of the case.*

Richard Hiltner: *I am thinking of Lilium tigrinum. I see a lot of moral problems—wanting to do the right thing—and then the sexual aspects. There are also some visual disturbances associated with Lilium tigrinum, and there is lasciviousness alternating with anger and this general rage and violence.*

Jonathan Shore: *I agree with Murray that Mercurius is an important thought for this case. What is interesting about the case from one angle is how much she holds it in and then throws herself against the doors. This would support the idea of a metal remedy. I also thought of Cuprum. Another thought would be Cenchris contortrix. She has this idea of wanting to hunt someone down, which suggests an animal remedy. There is a lot of anger. If we look at animal and snake remedies, we see that Cenchris is very big for dreams of rape.*

Judyth Reichenberg-Ullman: *I do not feel sure of the remedy. I thought a little about Lyssin and a lot about Hyoscyamus and Belladonna. However, I am wondering about the issue of when we should report somebody who comes to see us and talks about murdering people. My husband Bob had a patient who threatened to murder his ex-girlfriend. Bob actually did call the police after* *much agonizing. The police didn't do anything. About six months later we were told that this man had attempted to kill her, although he didn't succeed.*

Ohanian: *That is a good question. I am glad you brought it up. I was really worried that this woman would harm both herself and somebody else. I had my business manager call the local police department to see what responsibility we had and what we could do. They said that since she wasn't planning on killing one specific person that it was more in the psychological realm. They said to send her to a psychiatrist and to keep them posted. She already had a psychiatrist, with whom I spoke.*

What I did in this case was to have her call me every week. Every week we would touch base. We had a good relationship. I had known her a number of years and trusted that she would follow through with me.

Richard Pitt: *When I first looked at the case, I thought of Stramonium. You mentioned her history of being raped, so we have the etiology, the grief, the violence, the sexuality, and the waking as if from fright, which is a very strong symptom. She described hallucinations, violence, and evil feelings.*

But then Staphysagria also became very clear. I have certainly seen cases that seem to require Stramonium or Veratrum but that actually turn out to require Staphysagria. I feel more inclined toward Staphysagria because there is also a feeling of control, a quality of conscience there. This is sometimes found in Stramonium, but not so strongly. In Staphysagria, control is a prominent theme, and then they suddenly lose control and "snap." Also, the suicidal tendency by shooting is quite a strong Staphysagria tendency, for which it has been added to the repertory.

Helene Schwartzenberger: *When there is a rape and there is a possibility of having transmitted a syphilitic miasm, does this entirely change the person's constitution or do you have to give two types of remedies? When there is that overlay from an external source, how do you deal with that?*

Ohanian: *It is a good question. When she came in many years ago, with the herpetic symptoms, the Medorrhinum state seemed very clear, and it did, I believe, have a positive affect. It appears to have been an overlay from the previous rape. If it were the simillimum for the case, I don't think these other difficulties would have developed. I see the Medorrhinum as an overlay. I see* *an underlying remedy, the remedy I gave when she returned for treatment, which is, I believe, the simillimum.*

Analysis of Case Number 2

I thought about a number of remedies for this case: Medorrhinum, Anacardium, Staphysagria, Mercurius, and Hyoscyamus. First, I looked beyond the extreme obsessiveness in the case—to the fact that this very nice, somewhat meek, and mousy-appearing woman thought of nothing but raping, maiming, and murdering during most of her waking hours. Then I was able to see the strongest element in the case, which was the recurring hallucination and dream of dolls—voodoo dolls—stabbing or killing her. Considering the rubric, MIND, Delusions, sees devils, I probed further to see if I could confirm Anacardium:

I asked how she felt about herself inside. "I've felt evil in myself. I feel there are all sorts of demons inside. I live in this internal world that is so destructive. My therapist is out in the other world. It's so far away."

I asked about the voices she hears. She said they call her name just as she is going to sleep.

I asked her how she felt about herself growing up. "I think I'm stupid. I wasn't as quick as my brothers and sisters. I was dense, and I felt left out. I had a hard time in school. I didn't go to college. I couldn't think during exams. My mind would go blank. I'd fail, even though I studied hard."

So, given this information, I chose the following rubrics (Figure 3):

- MIND, Grief, ailments from.
- MIND, Kill, desire to.
- MIND, Suicidal disposition, shooting, by.
- MIND, Delusions, voices, hears, calling him.
- MIND, Delusions, devils, sees.
- MIND, Delusions, he is a devil.
- MIND, Delusions, he is separated from the world.

Plan: Anacardium 1M, single dose.

Analysis Options: Number of Rubrics, 25 polycrests

	Anac.	Stram.	Ant-c.	Hyos.	Med.	Op.	Plat.	Staph.
Total	7	5	4	6	4	4	5	8
Rubrics	6	4	3	3	3	3	3	3
MIND; AILMENTS from; grief	1	1	1	2		2	2	3
MIND; KILL, desire to	1	2		3	2	1	2	2
MIND; SUICIDAL disposition; shooting, by	1		2		1	1		3
MIND; DELUSIONS; calls; someone	1	1	1	1	1		1	
MIND; DELUSIONS; devils; he is a, that	1	1						
DELUSIONS; separated; world, from the, that he is	2							

Figure 3

Follow-Up on Case Number 2

Two Months After the Remedy

"I'm thinking more clearly now, although I still have trouble understanding what people are saying to me."

"Work is going great. I'm becoming more important there, more needed."

"I have a lot of physical energy."

"There's not a lot of rage now. I'm not having violent fantasies or dreams. I'm coming to terms. I'm not violent."

Complains of nausea and shakiness on rising for the past three weeks. Has to eat a cheese sandwich right away to feel better.

Herpes outbreak one week ago. Big sore. No prodrome.

Strong sexual desire.

Wants to be with a man in a loving relationship. (Currently in a lesbian relationship.)

Plan: Wait.

Four Months After the Remedy

She has a cold.

She had back spasm last week.

It's more difficult for her to think and understand people again.

Feeling guilty, dishonest.

Feeling pressured and pushed.

Her therapist wants her to see someone else to break transference. (The patient told her therapist about the violent fantasies toward the therapist, and the therapist was alarmed.)

She is thinking about shooting herself again.

Her violent thoughts are back.

Full of rage; taking risks while driving.

Assessment: Partial relapse. I did not want to wait for a full relapse.

Plan: Anacardium 30c, single dose.

Six Months After the First Remedy

"I'm more tolerant of myself since the remedy." She is much more tolerant of other drivers now and was able to be tolerant of an angry man at the grocery store.

"When my therapist cut me off I felt like a baby with no mother. That's the kind of desperation I felt inside."

She is working with a new therapist, learning to "be kind" to herself.

Her suicidal and violent feelings are much less.

Plan: Wait.

Eleven Months After the First Remedy

"I'm feeling really sharp mentally, like coming out of a psychosis. I feel fully healthy mentally. I took an IQ test and found out my IQ is 128 or higher. I'm really smart. I can do anything I want."

She is having more good feelings, and can express them easily.

More loving.

Her compassion for animals is returning. She wants to become a veterinarian.

She is angry (2) about how newborn lambs are treated. (She worked with them in a research setting.)

"I have all the care back, all the feelings I used to have. Now there is a lot of sadness, too."

"I feel more creative again. I'm composing music."

Her obsessiveness is considerably reduced.

Plan: Wait.

Thirteen Months After the First Remedy

"I feel good physically. I'm much more pleasant and productive."

"Violent thoughts haven't been a problem. Sometimes I get angry and want to take it out on a child abuser, but it isn't bad. I'm no longer in the mind set of a perpetrator.

Her obsessive sexual thoughts are gone.

"As soon as I had my grief over my therapist not being my mom, the sexual obsessions stopped. I'm finding myself feeling separate from others in a good way."

She no longer hears voices.

Plan: Wait.

Sixteen Months After the First Remedy

"I'm having more feelings like I used to, in my heart. I'm feeling more affection. I'm much more caring."

"I'm a lot stronger in speaking out and accepting other people's reactions. It's very hard when you speak out and others don't agree."

"The evil is gone. I don't even get irritated much anymore."

She had a bad herpes attack with her last menses.

Her sexual desire is way up.

She's lonely. Wants a lover.

Plan: Wait.

Twenty Months After the First Remedy

She is still doing quite well.

After a bodywork session, she had clear memories that her uncle had sexually abused her in childhood. She remembered that he had been a dollmaker and had frightened her with dolls. This helped her understand her hallucinations of voodoo dolls.

Three Years After the First Remedy

I called her up as I was preparing this presentation. She continues to do quite well in general. She said she had some dreams again of running from an attacker, but she faced the attacker and he went away. She no longer has the feeling that other people are better than she is. She said, "I just say what I see. I gave up that feeling that I never had anything to contribute and I never did anything right. I feel there has been a really big change inside me. I now have a certain amount of self-confidence that has staying power."

This is a fairly straightforward Anacardium case. It illustrates the elements of good and evil battling in a person, the extremely violent nature of the remedy, the strong sense of separation from the world, and the low level of self-confidence. We usually don't think of Anacardium with the etiology of symptoms coming on after grief, nor is it the first remedy we think of for obsessive-compulsive disorder. But it covers both these elements in this case very well, similar to the way Aurum muriaticum natronatum covered the obsessive-compulsive disorder in Case Number 1.

Other Aurum Muriaticum Natronatum and Anacardium Cases

Before I conclude, I want to mention two other confirmed cases of obsessive-compulsive disorder where Aurum muriaticum natronatum and Anacardium were used. The first is an Aurum muriaticum natronatum case. It involves a woman who as a child was sexually abused in a ritualistic way by family members. She had a great deal of grief about her family and about romantic relationships. Her obsession concerned a slight twinge of pain behind her sternum, a heaviness. She got to a point where she couldn't think about anything but this heaviness and, as a result, couldn't function in her daily life. By the time she came into the office she could hardly get out of bed. The remedy didn't cure the heaviness; it still comes and goes. It did, however, cure the obsessive thinking about it and the woman is carrying on with her life.

The second is an Anacardium case. A 45-year-old woman was obsessively concerned about meeting people. She was afraid of running into people she knew. She thought they were better than she and was afraid they'd think she was inept if she interacted with them. So, she got to the point where she wouldn't pick up her child at school, wouldn't go to the grocery store, and wouldn't shop in a neighborhood where an acquaintance lived. She would hardly go anywhere without being constantly on the lookout for a person she knew. She has had a couple of relapses over six years of treatment, but in general Anacardium has taken this symptom away and has allowed her to interact in the world without such limitation.

Karl Robinson: What were the indications for Anacardium in the last case you mentioned?

Ohanian: *She strongly lacked self-confidence and had a feeling of really wishing people harm. She is a very nice person, very meek and mild. She felt that if she tried to speak in a meeting she would come across as being a bumbler, someone who just didn't know anything. In addition, when she would have to go to a meeting, she would get so agitated that she would come home and curse at her family for hours. I interpreted her fear of meeting people as a fear of being evaluated or "tested."*

Anne Schadde, Heilprakterin

A CASE OF DEPRESSION AND LOSS OF JOY

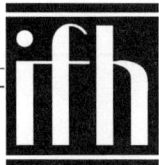

Anne Schadde began studying homeopathy in 1983 and has been practicing it since 1986. Before taking up homeopathy she was a secondary school teacher. She has been married for 26 years and has two sons, ages 25 and 22. Anne has studied with a variety of teachers. In 1992 she went to India to study with Rajan Sankaran, which was an important experience for her. In 1990 she co-founded the Homopathie-Forum in Munich and, in 1991, the European and International Councils for Homeopathy. "I am completely dedicated to homeopathy, always trying to develop my own access to the practice."

"The Highest Ideal of Cure"

Before I start with my presentation, I would like to share with you an insight that I got some months ago. The second passion in my life, after homeopathy, is psychology. In the last 25 years I have read many of Carl Gustav Jung's works. In one article he said, "In adolescence, when sexuality arises, the soul has been born." I asked myself what this means. How will the soul express itself? I have come to the conclusion that hobbies, the main interests between the ages of 12 and 16, express the soul. This is because hobbies express the first voluntary separation from one's parents. And the idea or the feeling behind the main interests from 12 to 16 years old continues throughout the whole life. Patients' hobbies will tell you more about them, regardless of their age, than any other symptom, especially in cases with emotional problems.

Now, what about me? How was it with me in my life? Well, during this period in my life I was interested in religion, praying, missionary work, and that sort of thing. And I still have a mission. That is why I must start with a paragraph from the *Organon* (paragraph 2):

> The highest ideal of cure is rapid, gentle and permanent restoration of the health, or removal and annihilation of the disease in its whole extent, in the shortest, most reliable, and most harmless way, on easily comprehensible principles.

What does Hahnemann mean by the "highest ideal of cure"? To me, "cure" in this paragraph applies to both the homeopath and the patient. The homeopath gets the chance to understand the patient on the deepest level we can perceive, to find the simillimum, and to eventually understand parts of the given remedy quite extensively. The patient gets what Hahnemann writes in paragraph 253: "...a greater degree of comfort, increased calmness and freedom of the mind, higher spirits—a kind of return of the natural state."

If there is a highest ideal, then there must be another possibility as well. Not every case can be solved according to Hahnemann's advice. Sometimes we don't find the correct remedy immediately; sometimes the remedy is not easy to see. Sometimes we have to go a long way in order to learn something. We stumble around, prescribe this and that, and finally have the chance to find the simillimum and to see a change in life.

The simillimum is a gift from God (to you and to the patient). With the simillimum patients are given the key for one part of their lives that has previously been locked. But this is not the end of the story. As it is said in fairy tales, "They live to the end of their life very happy and content...." Personal development never stops in life.

Let's go to the practical side of homeopathy. I am going to present two cases that required the same remedy. In the first case I will present video follow-ups over two years. This is a clear picture of a special remedy. Once you have seen it you will never miss it in the future. In the second case the picture is not as obvious. But you can see parts of the picture too. Unfortunately, I don't have video follow-ups of the second case. I interviewed the patient when I was in England, and we've been doing telephone follow-ups over the last two years. But it is interesting to see the same remedy in different shades.

When I interview patients I take everything into consideration: what they say, what they show, their clothes, their gestures, everything. Every little thing—even their names, their professions, their hobbies—can be important. "Can be" means only if it matches the center of the person, and then we can take it into consideration for the selection of the remedy.

I write down nearly every sentence the patient says. Their words are very good tools for studying materia medica. If the remedy is correct you can understand it through all the words people are saying, and this gives you a deep understanding of a remedy. And much more, it gives you the possibility of a deeper understanding of proving symptoms. Why do people say those things? What is meant by this symptom?

But I have to admit, it is very difficult to see a case in a foreign language, even with interpreters, because it is important to get the feeling when you listen to what people are saying. That's why in my simultaneous translation on the video I leave some gaps for you to get a feeling for the German language of the first patient.

Initial Visit

Male
Age 40

He runs his own driving school and is a driving instructor (car driving).

His father was an alcoholic, and the relationship between his parents was difficult.

When he was 19 years old, his father was nearly bankrupt and committed suicide. He is ashamed of his father's suicide. "This was wrong. One shouldn't do this."

Since then, he has experienced anxiety. "I have always had a lot of anxiety in the morning. I am scared of the coming day. My heart beats heavily with anxiety. I have to be very cautious, because this anxiety can take me over completely."

"In the evenings, after the day is over, I feel better. I am even enthusiastic in the evenings."

He worries about things that will happen to him. He worries about his economic situation. It is much worse in the morning.

He thinks about death a lot.

He has a feeling of fragility in his left foot, as if the bones were made of glass, as if he is standing directly with the bones on the floor. It is worse after a day of hectic activity; better when he is resting and in the evenings.

He sometimes sees a lump of mucus with his left eye, and he can't remove it.

As a child he had a croupy cough.

He often gets colds and influenzas.

The left side of his nose is always obstructed.

He is a very warm person, except in the belly region. He always has problems with his belly. It is a kind of coldness, ameliorated by warm bathing or a warm hand on the belly. In the morning he likes to hug his wife because of the coldness in this region.

He puts his feet out of his bed in the night.

He likes and craves fresh air. (When he comes to my clinic he always complains about my closed windows.)

He loves to eat. He is a gourmet. Likes knuckle of pork. He eats a lot. Craves meat. Salts everything a lot.

Averse to fat.

Loves beer (icy cold) and milk (icy cold).

He drinks a lot. He drinks one quart of beer in three gulps.

He has diarrhea in the morning and can't stand his own smell.

He can't stand tight clothes around his throat.

Suffers from recurrent styes on the eyelids, sometimes on the right and sometimes on the left side.

He retches every morning after rising.

He is very impatient and gets angry or irritated easily. Then he shouts at everybody. For example, if somebody turns right or left in a car without signalling, he gets angry and shouts even if he is alone in the car. "We have these rules and people have to behave correctly."

He is very efficient in everything he does. He came to the first interview with every symptom written down on a piece of paper. He is very careful.

Other examples of his efficiency: When he takes something from one room to another he likes to take everything with him so that he doesn't have to go twice, or when he goes shopping he has everything written down on a piece of paper. He never forgets anything. "This is a waste of time" he says, because he is always in a hurry while doing something.

He keeps all his things in order. He has a good system in his office.

He does not like to do useless things.

He likes to tell jokes. He is very witty, and likes teasing others.

His verbal expression is natural. He says everything as it is. Very open-minded.

Plan: Sulphur 200c, single dose.

Discovering the Simillimum

Third Visit: April 28, 1992

This is a video of the third time I saw him. So far, he has taken Sulphur and then a placebo. But after this third follow-up I knew the correct remedy.

[Editors' Note: The following is the transcript of the translation of the interview from German to English, as heard on the video. Dr. Schadde's comments are bracketed and italicized.]

> **Patient:** Everything is fine. My foot problems are gone. But the spot in my eye is still there. It is always there when I strain myself, when my body has to work harder than normal. Long highway drives in the night or so. I see it with one eye. It is a mucus lump. I cannot say it in another way. But it is only optically. There is something wrong in it. These are my only physical problems. In the morning I used to retch, mostly after my shower. I would retch with passion.
>
> **Schadde:** Any discharge?
>
> **Patient:** Nothing. Something is wrong with me. In the morning I am extremely hectic and irritable. I am a strange man in the morning. Now we come to the next point. Something is wrong in my brain. Fear, fear, fear in the morning. But in the evenings after the day is over I feel good. There is another thing I want to tell you. As you know, I had these black clouds in my mind. I miss the ease I had when I was 15 or 16, until my father's death. After the last remedy it was a little bit better, but now it is gone. I would like to have it back please. Not only this little bit. More please. For a short while I had the feeling it was a little bit better. But in the last months it has gotten worse rapidly.
>
> **Schadde:** How long was it better?

Patient: Very short. I don't know.

[Sulphur did something. His diarrhea in the morning, the styes, and the feeling in the bones have disappeared. He has no physical complaints. You saw the report he gave in the first minutes of the interview. In this stage we should never be satisfied with the result. The amelioration of the physical problems was only a kind of palliation. I don't say suppression because it didn't go deeper. The psychological problems that he has had for years have remained the same. That is why he came to me. And, when I saw that his deep problem was not better at all, I investigated again.]

Schadde: Tell me.

Patient: Nothing physically anymore. Perhaps my moaning and grumbling are a little bit better. For example, if somebody parks in the second line I can manage it a little bit better. But I am terribly unfair towards my wife. If my wife says something I go for her immediately. She is like a funnel. She has to swallow the whole shit. I know this mentally, but at that moment I lose my control. Shit.

Schadde: What kind of problems are these?

Patient: Tiny little things: uncleaned shoes, no fresh pants, wrong socks together, I cannot find my cup. I am a "Tüpferlscheißer" (fusspot) with the others; not with myself.

["Tüpferlscheißer" (fusspot) is a very funny word in German. I looked it up in the dictionary. It means he is critical even about the tiniest things.]

Patient: When we talked on the phone I told you my physical complaints were better. I am always in a hurry. I feel like blocking somebody's way. It is terrible for me if something is not flowing.

I'm telling you a lot of rubbish!

I like fresh air and when the wind is blowing. I would have opened all those windows. Air. I like it when there is fresh air.

Schadde: What do you like to eat?

Patient: Everything. Italian food. Meat. Things with garlic. I don't like vegetables. This is rather something for milk-giving animals. You know, it is my bad luck that I like everything. Well, I don't like fat—only pork meat—but not the wobbly fat. Only the crust.

At the age of 16 or 17 you could discover everything without sorrows. Highlights. Super-pleasure. Life was fun. Life was easy without sorrows. No worries. Fun inside. Life was great. Nothing special. No sorrows. I would like to have it back. It is like fresh air for the soul, like thoughts getting to a breezy place on a meadow somewhere.

[*Here, he mentions a symptom on the mental level that he has on the physical level. To me, this is a very important symptom because we have the confirmation on another level.*]

Patient: One thing I want to say is that I am very capricious. I'm up one minute and down the next—very suddenly. And it is different; sometimes things bother me and sometimes not. Very quick. In the mornings I tend to be nasty. Under the shower I grumble, thinking that I'll write a letter of complaint to someone or I'll go there and kick him or throw him over the fence. If I don't take care, I get stuck in my anger. Or when I am waiting for an answer to a letter, I stand under the shower and think, "Damned person. Why doesn't she answer?" It's as if I am searching for somebody I can attack.

[*This is very interesting. On the one hand he is a very polite and orderly person, but on the other hand he can be angry and impolite.*]

Patient: My shirt doesn't fit; it's too tight. I closed the last button only because it is polite. I like to have my shirt open. After the last remedy it was itching and I sat there like a monkey. But it was gone after one week.

The worst thing in my life is when my wife tells me on the phone that we have received an official letter—from the tax office, from the district court, or so—and she cannot or will not open the letter. My whole day is spoiled; I am finished. Even if it would be better to wait, I must solve the problem immediately—even if I lose money or anything. For example, I'd never forget the date of a trial—not out of respect—but I couldn't ignore it. "One should not do this."

Tardiness. This is the worst thing. I drive like crazy just to be on time. I am always on time. I cannot bear to be ten seconds late, and I realize immediately if you are ten seconds late.

I am a pedant.

If I don't like somebody, I will tell him immediately.

What a lot you're writing down! But, yes, it is your work.

[*Here you see more of the same. He is very intolerant to everybody. When I first saw him the patient who had been scheduled before him had canceled the appointment. So I was waiting for him. When I picked him up from the waiting room he said, "I said to my wife, if I have to wait too long I will go."*

I try not to get angry with a patient in such a situation. He's doing me a favor by giving me a clear picture of his state. If you get angry with the patient then you start to react—exactly what you are not supposed to do. We need to be "vorurteilsfreie Beobachter," unprejudiced observers, as Hahnemann calls it. So I immediately started thinking. "What is this? Is this haughtiness, impatience, or feeling hurried?" This is what I have to find out. Then, if other things the patient says fit together, at least I understand a part of the story.

In my experience, your best understanding of a patient comes without asking, just by observing and understanding what is said incidentally. These are the most important clues. I always try to understand what they mean and what the reasons are for saying those things. This means the patients have to guide me into their own story. I don't know their story better than they do. But I have the advantage that I am not stuck in the story (not yet!). That is why I can be more objective and see things clearer.

Let me tell you just a short story. Months ago my assistant, who takes the preliminary information from new patients, came out of the waiting room and gave me a new patient's card. I looked into her face and said to her, "What has happened to you? You look so overwhelmed." She said, "Yes. It was quite a strange situation. While I was taking the address, the new patient, a very strong woman, kept putting me down. I had to take care that she didn't stampede me into doing something totally different than what I wanted." I asked, "How do you feel?" She said, "I feel as if she tried to trick me. She was very clever but very polite. I was totally confused and tried to control the situation."

You see, this was the first information about the unconscious of both people involved. Sometimes you can use it for the selection of the remedy, and sometimes not. Hahnemann tells us not to be prejudiced. I didn't search for a remedy at this point. But after I took the case I realized that the remedy was already quite clear after this small incident. It was Lachesis.

We have to be aware of every little situation and every symptom. But we can repertorize the story only if we can confirm these things with other pieces of the puzzle. What is the meaning of "the totality of symptoms"? The correct remedy will seldom come out if we put all the symptoms together in the computer and wait for the answer. I try to avoid the word "never," because coincidentally it can come out. But if you don't know what you are doing and something comes out that is out of your control, you don't learn anything. This is a double blind. The computer doesn't know what you are doing—as far as I know—and you don't know what the computer is doing.

Homeopathy is not an algorithm. It will always be the understanding of the human mind through another human mind. The computer is only a tool to give you hints, but nobody else can understand the patient better than you. The patients come to you at one point in their lives. Homeopathy is a "healing art." To produce art every homeopath has to be an artist. We must be an artist in understanding the individuality of a person and what fits together in the symptomatology, in the behavior, in the language, in the life story, in the chosen profession, and so on. **The totality of the symptoms must be everything that fits into the whole picture of the person.** *Only this gives the hint for the correct remedy. This is my understanding.*]

> **Dolfy Freinquel:** *I was thinking about Magnesia carbonica. I will try to go in order: anxiety in the morning, feeling better in the evening, sticking his feet out of bed, diarrhea in the morning, desire for milk, desire for open air, aversion to vegetables, and the lump of mucus in the left eye. I prescribed this remedy just once, and I am not sure if the essence looks different from what I saw. If Magnesia carbonica is the right remedy, then I will tell a story.*
>
> *I also noticed his involvement with himself. He is very aware of what is happening, what he is thinking, and what is around him—his shoes, his cup, and all those things.*
>
> **Guy Kokelenberg:** *I thought about Medorrhinum, because of the mucus in his eyes, the evening amelioration, and the anxiety in the morning. He has a sort of anxiety if the time is set. There is the coldness of his abdomen. "Coldness in external abdomen" is Medorrhinum. And he has a desire for beer, although for Munich people this is not a symptom (audience laughter)!*
>
> **Schadde:** *Especially for a Bavarian (audience laughter).*

Audience: Exactly. However, I don't think of Medorrhinum as being a "fusspot."

Schadde: No. This was one of the reasons I chose the particular remedy for him.

Kokelenberg: Other symptoms for Medorrhinum include the difficult respiration, wanting to be fanned, wanting freedom in his mind, too, not wanting to be involved, and sticking his feet out.

Suzanne Adams: I was wondering about Sulphuric acid. I don't know much about the remedy, but it is hurried, has a cold stomach, has anxiety in the morning, is worse from heat, is critical, is impatient, and desires fresh air. He seemed very Sulphur-like to me.

Analysis

Now let's try to understand what we've got in this case. Which symptoms fit into the whole picture of the patient? What is the main impression you get? He is a person with charisma. He says everything with a kind of passion. It is not only interesting what people say but also how they say it.

On the other hand he can be quite aggressive. I would say abusive. But be cautious. This is part of his passion too. Whatever he is, does, or says, he always reacts in the same way: when he tells about the food he likes, when he tells about driving in streets and somebody behaving incorrectly, when he tells about his anxiety, when he explains the feeling in his youth, even when he describes how it would be if I opened my windows. *Passion* is the background for his reaction. So we've already got one of the first symptoms, because we can see it running through the whole case: MIND, Passionate.

I guess nobody will ever tell you that they are passionate. We have to see this or understand this in the whole story—in every sentence, in each reaction.

And what else do we have? When he talks he explains everything in flowery terms. He doesn't say it with one sentence. Here we can use the rubric, MIND, Loquacity, cheerful.

He is a very nice man. He tells jokes all the time. It is a shame that you couldn't understand the German. In nearly every statement he jokes about himself. He calls himself a "fusspot." Bavarian people can be like this, very witty, and they joke about themselves. We can use the rubric, MIND, Jesting.

Better yet, if we combine both symptoms, we can use the rubric, MIND, Loquacity with jesting.

Then let's take one more symptom with expressions on more than one level: GENERALITIES, Air, open, desire for. He explained this on two levels. He first mentioned his desire to open the windows in my office. And then he mentioned his emotional problem, "It is like fresh air for the soul, like thoughts getting to a breezy place on a meadow somewhere."

If we repertorize now, the remedy must be Kali iodatum (Figure 1). Let's look into some very interesting rubrics that list Kali iodatum:

- MIND, Abusive, family and children. (He said he was unfair to his wife; she has to swallow the whole "shit.") Or MIND, Unfeeling, hard-hearted with his family.

- MIND, Fear, dawn, of the return of. (The original symptom in Allen's materia medica is as follows: "He dreads the return of dawn, and the most trivial details of daily life seem insupportable to him." In the morning he is scared about how to manage the day. It is very important to note that during the whole interview he talks about the shower in the morning. What is said in this symptom, "...again a new day." What are the most trivial details?)

- MIND, Irritability, with sadness. (He expressed this when he said that it is actually fear. This means a kind of depression, which is the reason why he is so angry.) Or MIND, Sadness, mental depression, with irritability.

As I said before, I prefer to see the original symptoms in the materiae medicae in order to understand the remedy. Let's look a little bit deeper. We can clearly see the miasmatic background. It must be a remedy with a high syphilitic tendency (which Kali iodatum is). Why? For these reasons:

- Father committed suicide.
- Pain in the bones (deep in the bones).
- Depression when the day is beginning.
- Hot-warm person with a desire for open air.
- Problems with eyes.

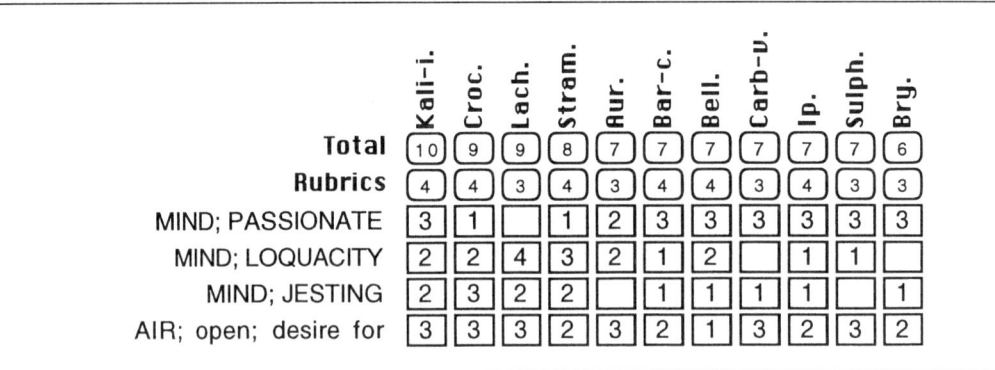

	Kali-i.	Croc.	Lach.	Stram.	Aur.	Bar-c.	Bell.	Carb-v.	Ip.	Sulph.	Bry.
Total	10	9	9	8	7	7	7	7	7	7	6
Rubrics	4	4	3	4	3	4	4	3	4	3	3
MIND; PASSIONATE	3	1		1	2	3	3	3	3	3	3
MIND; LOQUACITY	2	2	4	3	2	1	2		1	1	
MIND; JESTING	2	3	2	2		1	1	1	1		1
AIR; open; desire for	3	3	3	2	3	2	1	3	2	3	2

Figure 1

Plan: Kali iodatum 1M, single dose.

Follow-Up After the Kali Iodatum

May 1992

Telephone interview.

In the past month since he took the Kali iodatum all his symptoms, which had disappeared during the period he was taking Sulphur, have come back:

- Diarrhea in the morning on waking.
- Coldness in his belly.
- Pain in the bones of his foot (has to put his feet out of the bed).
- Stye in the left eyelid twice.
- Impatient with "the whole world."
- "Up one minute and down the next."

He is very angry about the return of the symptoms and criticizes me. Says that I must have made a mistake.

"I feel like a car that is standing still and somebody is trying to drive it at full throttle."

[With this sentence he describes exactly where he is stuck. I will try to explain it later. I calmed him down and told him to wait, that everything will disappear soon. Until his next visit ten

months later I heard about his condition only indirectly through his wife and his son, who are under my treatment.]

March 23, 1993

I saw him eleven months after taking the remedy. He didn't come voluntarily. I asked him because I wanted to get the video follow-up. He felt very good and didn't see any reason to see me.

> **Patient:** Actually I didn't realize that it was better. I would realize it only when I thought I had to phone you or when my wife asked me how I felt.
>
> But when I look back I get the insight that this is exactly what I wanted to get back. The feeling of being free, like flashes of lightning, as when I was 15 or 16. Free as a bird. Not as serious.
>
> Life is much easier now, I don't have any problems. I don't get upset even if somebody is double-parked.

[*This is what Hahnemann writes in paragraph 253: "...a greater degree of comfort, increased calmness and freedom of the mind, higher spirits—a kind of return of the natural state."*]

> **Patient:** Sometimes I call someone a dirty bastard. But it is okay. Really good.
>
> **Schadde:** You didn't get this with any previous remedy?
>
> **Patient:** At the beginning, I told my wife that I had to go to a psychiatrist because I thought something was wrong in my mind. I was scared about how I could get through the day. I felt anguish about how I would give the theory lectures in my school. I was afraid I would lose the thread while speaking.
>
> I can handle my students easier now; I'm not as aggressive anymore.
>
> I am calmer now, and more sympathetic. It doesn't hurt me if somebody does something that disturbs me.

I feel considerably easier. I laugh at anybody who challenges me.

I mean it is really like cheekiness. For example, I went to a bank for a mortgage for my house and they wanted to take a picture of the house. One morning the man from the bank came at 10 a.m. without an appointment. I was still in my pajamas and refused. He said, "It's you who wants the mortgage." And I said, "But it's you who earns money with me."

Schadde: You wouldn't have done this before?

Patient: Never. I would have said to myself, "It is impossible. You can't do this." Now I behave as if I am the emperor.

I feel really good.

I would never have thought that this tiny little pill could have such an effect. I thought I had to do something myself. With painkillers you realize the effect. You get a little bit numb in your head. (Some people are always numb in their head.) But with this pill I didn't even realize what was happening.

[*This is a very important sentence. Nietzsche says, "Now I know that you are cured. Healthy is only this person who forgets." In the next follow up he repeats it again and again.*]

December 16, 1993

Patient: Here in my mind everything is fine. My fear is gone. No problems anymore. I am nasty sometimes in traffic. But, you know, I have to drive the whole day.

Schadde: Tell me, when?

Patient: If somebody double-parks and I have to wait in order to pass him.

Schadde: Is there any difference from the past?

Patient: My financial fears are gone. Nothing disturbs or burdens me anymore. That's why I was very astonished that I have to come to you. I began to think this morning, when my wife told me that we have an appointment, that with the best will in the world I cannot find anything that should be repaired.

Schadde: You came only because I wanted the follow-up?

Patient: I feel excellent. But my condition went away very gradually. I didn't even realize. It is a difference like day and night. But, when I look back, I know that I had this fear.

I drink two to four cups of coffee a day.

Schadde: Any dreams?

Patient: Yes. I dream, but I forget immediately. People from my childhood, from my school days, or from my time in the military, but nothing special. What I dream I forget immediately after the shower.

[*This is what I realized quite a few times in cases like this. Their dreams are filled with people from childhood, or people they haven't seen for years, or events from childhood. It is as if the unconscious tries to go back and remind them of stories from the old days. Dreams are codings from the unconscious, and our task is to decipher them. In some cases dreams have brought up interesting subjects. It is important not to stop with the treatment at this point. You are not only a doctor. You are a psychologist as well. Health is not a state. It is a process, most of all a process of handling one's unconscious. "Know thyself" is said on the steps to the temple of Delphi and not "Be free of symptoms and lead a happy life." That's why I go on working with patients at those periods in their life when a remedy induces movement from their unconscious.*]

Patient: There's nothing wrong with me anymore. The problems I had, such as the tender foot, are gone. It is different now. I have an easy time.

It changed imperceptibly.

I get along with people easier if I want. This is a remarkable difference. I'm remarkably better.

I knew mentally that these things shouldn't be like that. It was not necessary to get scared about all those things, but on the level of my feeling I was completely stuck.

I am not musical, but I connect Bavaria, beer garden, Oktoberfest, everything that is beautiful with the "Trumpet Echo." A zest for life I would say.

[*The "Trumpet Echo" is his favorite piece of music. But we can't use the rubric, Desire for music. Here we have to understand why he likes it. As you know, Kali people have a deep connection to family. "They need their support," Rajan Sankaran says. What does "family" mean? It means people who are related by blood or, in a former time, have the same name. Let's extend this definition. The wider family could be the country, for example, or the region, the religion, the culture, people who speak the same language. Wherever we feel secure and at home. And this patient has a deep connection to Bavaria. Munich is the capital of Bavaria. Bavaria is different from the rest of Germany. The people speak a special dialect; they have special weather (we call it Föhn); they have a special culture; and they love beer gardens.*]

Another Kali Iodatum Case

Male
Age 46

This is the case of an Irish man. The quality of the video is not that high because of the light. He is different from the first man. He is not as passionate, but there is some similarity.

Initial Visit

Chief Complaint: A very painful fissure in the anus.

He had the fissure cauterized five years ago.

It is aggravated by heat, such as a warm car seat. It is ameliorated by cold applications.

High blood pressure.

Dyslexia. Cannot spell correctly—numbers and letters. He never writes.

At first he was very embarrassed to talk about his symptom, but this disappeared very quickly.

He is always busy. Very restless and talkative.

No fear. "All your fears are gone if your morale is rising."

It is hard for him to get angry. "I am the person who keeps talking all the time."

He eats a lot. Desires fat, potatoes, bacon, meat, and eggs.

Averse to fish.

Cannot stand tight things around his neck. He calls it claustrophobia.

Cannot stand the summer heat; feels better in winter.

(Video excerpts were shown.)

Analysis

Here is one of the main features of Kali people. He tries to be very correct. You see it in his answers. He always wears trousers with creases, even when he is not working. He has been unemployed for three years, and I assume he doesn't want to work in this occupation anymore (MIND, Business, averse to). His hair is very tidy, with a very stiff part.

I lived in his house for a time, so I knew that he had very strict rules. But he is a wonderful person, very polite and very nice. He is not as witty as the patient in Case Number 1, but he is very loquacious, very quick-witted.

He is a Catholic. He goes to church every Sunday, even though his wife is not religious at all. He is very fond of his family (Kali element). This is what you can understand of Kali people. They are very loyal people (to the church, to the family). They stick to you once they have chosen you.

He does not show anger; he is too polite to show his anger. But deep inside there is a lot of anger, controlled anger.

I looked into the rubric, RECTUM, Anus, fissure, and I saw Kali iodatum. I also looked at his amelioration from cold water, and his aggravation from heat, even a warm car seat. I connected all the things I observed, plus the miasmatic background (son has a spina bifida and is in a wheelchair), and eventually I got the remedy: Kali iodatum.

The Central Themes of Kali Iodatum

Let's divide Kali from iodatum in order to understand both. We all have learned from former teachers that Kali people are conservative. Their main theme is morality: what is right; what is wrong. (Remember what a terrible deed it was to double-park in Case Number 1!) Why are they conservative? Who needs to have right and wrong? Who needs rules? Who needs the support of a group?

We always get the answer from the provings, from our materiae medicae. One main theme in Kali is weakness. The spinal column is affected. Pain and weakness. And if your back is weak, the whole body is weak and this creates a feeling of fragility. If you don't have support you can easily get hurt. The more support you get, the better you can stand. That's why rules are very important. You have somebody who tells you what is right and wrong.

Do you remember what the first patient said about the bones in his foot? They feel fragile after a hectic day, as if made from glass. In the repertory we find only Thuja for this symptom. But the understanding of the fragility in Thuja is different. It is the "delusion that body and soul are separated" that creates the fragility of Thuja. And if you have only one part available, you become fragile and easily hurt. You have to cover up in order to survive.

But this is totally different from the Kali fragility. Kali people need support; when they are alone they feel fragile. And in Case Number 1 everything started after his father's suicide. He didn't have any support, even if he were very able to manage his own life. But the delusion stayed the same. In each life everybody gets hurt more or less at one point. To know that somebody was hurt and what it was that hurt this person doesn't lead you anywhere. The wound itself is not important. For us it is only important to understand how people *react* to the injuries in their lives. And he reacted in the Kali iodatum way.

In Kali iodatum the iodatum element is very prominent. They are restless. They are on the move. Dromomania. The impulse to run. You know the rubric? And for being on the move you need food, don't you? For iodatum, eating is very important. They have the compulsive idea that they are going to starve. And, if you run and run, you get hot. The iodatum burns and burns and is better with cold applications. These are the main elements in iodatum. From these elements we can understand the core. They have to live life. Eating is very important. Motion is necessary. Talking is very important. (Isn't talking the motion of the mouth?) Loquacity is oral satisfaction, like cigarettes or pacifiers.

The first patient said, "I feel like a car that is standing still and somebody is trying to drive it at full throttle." After taking Kali iodatum he said one sentence that explains the remedy quite clearly. "The door was locked, and the remedy could open it."

What is typical for Kalium iodatum? They can be entertainers. They are very witty, quick-witted, social, sympathetic. (The first patient telephoned me one day to ask whether I could help one of his students who was totally depressed. He couldn't bear to see this anymore; he felt so sorry for him.) On the other hand, they can be very irritable and abusive to the family and to everyone else.

Kali iodatums have to cool themselves down. Clarke writes, "Irresistible desire for the open air; walking in open air does not fatigue." Heat, hot weather, and warm rooms aggravate their symptoms.

In the materiae medicae it is said under Kali iodatum, "excessively thin." This does not fit either person in the cases I just presented. The first patient goes in the opposite direction. But "to be thin" is a very important symptom of iodatum. So, what is the value of confirmatory symptoms? Which symptoms do we really need? Hahnemann explains the problem in paragraph 156 "...for it is next to impossible that medicine and disease should cover one another symptomatically as exactly as two triangles with equal sides and equal angles...."

How can we handle the problem practically? My proposal for these situations is that if I can understand the center of the patient as deeply as I am able to and if I try to understand the provings and symptoms in the same way, then I don't need to have all the confirmatory symptoms.

Where confusion about the confirmatory symptoms begins, the process of deep understanding often starts. At this point you will have to leave the beaten track of agglomerated symptoms and start to understand the central idea of the case. This, and not just profound knowledge of materia medica, is what Hahnemann meant in his motto "aude sapere." This motto is taken from Horace's "epistolae" (letters). The German philosopher Kant translated it to mean, "Have the courage to use your own mind." This should still be homeopathy's maxim today.

Karl Robinson: *I want to thank you very much for broadening my understanding of family to include the language, culture, and country. That was very enlightening to me because I have always thought of family quite narrowly. If you can say anything more about that, I would appreciate it.*

Schadde: *For me, the family consists of the people who belong to you. You feel you belong to them, and, when they leave you, you feel very alone, very forsaken. This is part of the Kali story. This includes one's country, as you could especially see in the first case. I have seen this in many Kali cases.*

The family is very important to Kali, even if he—as it is said in the materiae medicae—"quarrels with his bread and butter." That is why he quarrels, because he needs them. We often have to understand the opposite side. Why do people act like this? When they quarrel, it is not because they don't like who they are quarreling with. You quarrel with people you like. If you don't have any connection to them, forget it.

You can see this lack of connection in Natrum muriaticum cases, for example. They don't quarrel that often with others, because they do not have a deep connection to others. It is just a one-to-one relationship. They are withdrawn.

Kali people quarrel because they need the person, they need the country. These are the people who sit in environmental parties and fight for their surroundings; they fight for everything. This is what I have observed in my practice.

Ahmed Currim: *Did you say that you have Kali iodatum listed for fissures of the rectum?*

Schadde: *Yes. It is in the Complete Repertory.*

Ahmed Currim: *Also, I just want to point out that Iodum is listed in the repertory under obesity.*

Nancy Herrick: *In the first case, his father committed suicide and there was the sense of being betrayed (Iodum) by the one he put his trust in, his family (Kali). This was a big factor that influenced his whole life, and that fits the Kali iodatum theme (as described by Sankaran).*

Schadde: *Yes. He felt totally forsaken. He told me in the first interview that he could not understand why his father would leave him. One should never do this, to have a son at the age of 19 and leave him.*

Nancy Herrick: Right. It illustrates the morality issue as well as the betrayal issue. Thank you for a beautiful case.

Helene Schwartzenberger: I have two questions with regard to the rubrics, Forsaken (abandoned) and Loquacity. I have had several discussions with other homeopaths about this. I agree with the way you have interpreted them. It is my feeling, first of all, that sometimes a rubric is not exactly a symptom and that sometimes it is. It is hard sometimes to differentiate when to consider it a symptom and when not to. Sometimes the feeling of being forsaken is real, not a delusion, and sometimes the feeling of being abandoned is a delusion. You have to look into which is which. In this case, it didn't necessarily seem to be a delusion. It was real. It was an abandonment on one level, and there was a sense of forsakenness. I suspect we should think more of the Kali remedies for the forsaken feeling.

With regard to loquacity, I remember hearing another lecturer say that unless the loquacity is pathological, he wouldn't consider it as a symptom for the case. The loquacity in these cases didn't seem so pathological. I would like to understand how you decided to use loquacity as a symptom.

I also would like you to elaborate to some extent on the other Kali remedies and how they have this attachment to family and the broader sense of family.

Schadde: We should put every remedy in the forsaken rubric because most diseases start after this sort of experience. That is why I never look in the rubric, Forsaken feeling, because, as I said earlier, the reaction to the injury and to the hurt is what is important, not the wound itself. This is a very important point.

Loquacity is motion of the mouth, as I said before. You start to be loquacious to calm down your inner feeling, as we could see in the first case. That is why I said he reacted to the injury, to the wound itself, in a Kali iodatum way. Kali iodatum reacts with loquacity. You can see this in the repertory: Loquacious with jesting. Only three or four remedies are in this rubric.

To talk about all the other Kali remedies would simply require more time than we have.

Sheryl Kipnis, ND, DHANP,
and Stephen King, ND, DHANP

A SMALL
BUT USEFUL
REMEDY

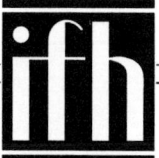

Sheryl Kipnis is a graduate of the National College of Naturopathic Medicine. She has practiced homeopathy in Seattle since 1982 and is co-founder of the Ravenna Homeopathic Clinic. Sheryl has been an instructor in the IFH Professional Course since 1985. She is board-certified in homeopathy by the Homeopathic Academy of Naturopathic Physicians (HANP) and is a past member of the HANP board of directors. She is the proud mother of one-year-old Hanna Simona Kipnis King.

Stephen King is a graduate of the National College of Naturopathic Medicine. He has practiced homeopathy in Seattle since 1982 and is co-founder of the Ravenna Homeopathic Clinic. Stephen has been an instructor in the IFH Professional Course since 1984 and is past president of the IFH board of directors. He is board-certified in homeopathy by the Homeopathic Academy of Naturopathic Physicians.

Introduction

We all have the tendency to see only what is familiar. But once we have seen something for the first time, it is much easier to recognize it the second time. One of the great values of these case conferences is that we get to benefit from each other's "first times" with lesser known remedies.

We are going to present two cases, and describe a third, all helped by the same remedy. It is a remedy that neither of us had any experience with until we saw it for the first time, and then it was much easier to recognize it when it came along again. Our intent is to give you some basic and central ideas about this remedy and to show what it might look like in different people.

We'll present both cases first and then we'll discuss the analyses and follow-ups.

Presentation of Case Number 1
(Dr. Kipnis)

Female
Age 41

Initial Visit: December 8, 1992

Two concerns: Low energy; depression.

She believes her lack of energy may be related to her 22-month-old child. "Still a pull
of energy from me to her. She takes a lot of physical and psychic energy from me."

She is still nursing the child morning and evening.

She often does not feel rested in the morning, despite eight hours of solid sleep.

Observation: Pronounced swelling and dark red, purplish circles beneath her eyes.

After the birth of her child she took a year-long break from her work.

She likes to work (2). Thrives on working hard; "110 percent."

Has worked in politics for many years.

Over the last 15 years she has experienced cyclic periods of depression without cause.
About one year ago she was working half time and therefore had time to focus on
herself. She went into psychotherapy, which she ended three months ago because
she wasn't getting much out of it. During the therapy she looked into her family,
childhood, and other possible causes but could find no cause for the depression. She
describes her childhood as idyllic and trouble-free. She is the oldest of two sisters,
and describes her parents as easygoing and complacent. Therefore, she believes the
depression is chemical. She thinks it may be cyclic on a monthly basis—PMS.

She and her husband were in therapy five years ago and found it very helpful.

Her menses is due in a few days.

Since last Friday she has been feeling impatience and rage very close to the surface (2).
(She is smiling and cheerful as she says this.)

It takes very little to set her off. She becomes mean-spirited (2), wanting to kick the cat (doesn't actually do this), and is impatient with her child.

Her mother has unacknowledged bouts of depression.

She and her mother both present an upbeat persona.

She mistrusts therapy. "Their whole shtick is to keep you coming back."

Generally, she is very self-analytical (2). "Translates into self-consciousness." (Sighs.)

Feels overwhelmed with choices, having to make decisions. Wants to shut down. Feels overloaded. This is a paradox because her work has always been demanding and she feels happiest when it is that way.

At one point about five or six years ago, after much overwork, she had severe pain in her abdomen (3). It was diagnosed as gastritis, which was relieved with Tagamet. It recurred within one year, but she hasn't had it since.

When asked about her tendency to do several things at once she replies, "That is a complete understatement! I get really impatient with people who do only two things at once!"

Feels a complete and total lack of peace (3). Just wants to leap back into action so she can feel some purpose (2).

When she is down, life as a whole feels meaningless (2).

She is never suicidal. "It feels like an existential crisis."

When working 110 percent there's no time for paralysis. But right now she cannot escape in her work.

When she is in this state she becomes more upbeat with friends and colleagues. "A real mask."

Her family and husband get the brunt of it. "I'm short-tempered (2), irrational. I can explode (2), start yelling (2), or just be cold and ignoring. 'Leave me alone.'"

Feels like screaming and yelling, but doesn't.

Makes biting comments (2); is intolerant (2).

No destructive behavior; just feels like doing it.

Her energy feels "mired down."

Previously, if she was feeling really down she would run for a long distance to feel better (2). But she can't do this now because of her child.

She has been with her husband for 18 years; married eight years.

She had abortions at 23 and 33 years old. She and her husband had no intention of having children, she in particular. At 36 years old she was reconsidering having children and then got pregnant before she had made the decision. Miscarried around eight weeks and then made a firm decision to have children.

She became pregnant again at age 37 and had a missed abortion around eight weeks. Went to a fertility specialist who diagnosed luteal phase defect and inadequate progesterone. Was treated with progesterone.

Her last pregnancy was easy; she was able to continue working. The pregnancy went two weeks post-term and was induced. Had a cesarean section due to fetal distress.

Feels that whatever she is doing is never enough (2).

Needs to do something that is socially conscious, meaningful to her, and useful. "I want to be more than just a cog in the wheel."

She has a history of overextending herself (2) when working.

She never has to look for a job. Always gets hired away from what she is doing.

When she is feeling down she wonders, "Is this the most important thing I can be doing right now?" (2).

Searches for meaning (2).

She is not generally fearful. Afraid of caves (1) and horror movies (2). Conjures up images from the movies later at night when alone, and then becomes irrational (2).

Loves to be outside. Rock climbing is her very favorite activity in life (3). Starts imagining all sorts of possibilities when she's climbing.

She is not especially sympathetic and tends to be judgmental (2). Judges friends for not doing what they say they want, even her best friends.

She sees pictures of starving kids and doesn't want to feed them; wants to work on population control.

Ran for a political office once in another state. Didn't win but loved every aspect of doing it.

Her menses are regular and light. She is not sure her moods are really linked to her menstrual cycle. But in the last few months she has noticed that she feels bad the week before her menses and then feels better ("relief from pressure") once the flow starts.

Feels warm (2). Not much tolerance for heat. Very cranky (2) in summer.

(Her cheeks are red.) In response to my question about her red cheeks she says she is aware that they feel hot and that this is neither common nor unusual for her.

Has Wolff-Parkinson-White Syndrome, a condition of the heart that causes tachycardia. Diagnosed 15 years ago when she was experiencing chest pain, which she thought was heartburn. Occurs infrequently and irregularly. Can be triggered by anaerobic exercise. Heart beats more than 180 beats per minute.

No other physical complaints.

Her sexual desire is almost nonexistent right now (2). She thinks it has to do with having a child. She and her husband used to have sex in the afternoon or on weekends, and the opportunities are fewer with a child around. Her sexual desire was average before having a child. Sex is almost always pleasurable for her.

She didn't want children because she felt there were plenty of children in the world. "It was selfish. I didn't want to spend the time and energy on a child."

When she was around 35 years old she saw lots of older people around her and realized there would be no regeneration if younger people didn't have children.

She thought she could get her "kid fix" from others but realized she couldn't.

She sometimes feels resentful about having a child. But mostly feels fine about it. "It's an interesting, wonderful experience, and I'm getting a lot out of it."

Her appetite, digestion, and elimination are normal.

No food cravings.

Averse to sauerkraut (1) and fat.

She isn't thirsty (2). Has to force herself to drink.

She generally feels best at night (2). "When the day is over there are no more expectations of me (2). I can relax and become really productive."

She drags out of bed in the morning (2). Takes a while to wake up.

Averse to sleeping on her back. Rarely salivates in her sleep; once or twice a month.

Her relationship with her husband is good. They have very separate lives. She didn't tell him she was coming here.

She didn't marry for a long time because there weren't any marriages she wanted to emulate. Her husband feared she would leave at any time, so she agreed to get married but restated her lack of desire for children.

Presentation of Case Number 2
(Dr. King)

Female
Age 50

Initial Visit: May 5, 1993

Chief Complaint: She has a lifelong history of bowel problems. Has had a nervous stomach since childhood, and intermittent diarrhea, hemorrhoids, and yeast vaginitis from adolescence to her mid-40s. Has suffered from chronic constipation (2) alternating with diarrhea for many years.

(Her cheeks are red.)

"I have been blessed with good health and a good constitution."

After a brief marriage at age 21 she developed severe diarrhea, which would come on soon after eating. Now, in recent years, the diarrhea comes when she waits too long to eat.

"I can go a long time without eating. My body can take a lot of abuse."

Her stools are hard (2), small (2), and incomplete. She skips days.

She still gets hemorrhoids occasionally.

Sometimes when she is sleeping on her abdomen, she wakes with burning pain in the abdomen.

She had chronic tonsillitis as a child. Her tonsils and adenoids were removed when she was 16 years old.

Her mother has had irritable bowel syndrome and constipation for many years.

"I can work hard for others, but not so easily for myself."

She has a layer of self-doubt. Asks recurrent questions about what she knows. Does she know enough?

She had a vision that she knew all conventional and alternative medicine.

"I seem very confident, yet a part of me is uncertain."

"I am intense, impatient, critical, and judgmental. I can be anxious, kind of obsessive, especially about work."

"I am not a workaholic anymore. There is less 'doing' than before."

She went to chiropractic school when she was a single mother with a young child, "and it kept on from there."

Has a tendency to get low back pain, which began in 1964 (age 22) while working at a sedentary job. She has had back pain on and off for a long time. In the early 1980s it became very bad, with pain in the lower right lumbar and in the left neck. X-rays showed that she had six instead of five lumbar vertebrae and that there were long transverse processes in the cervical vertebrae. The pain was relieved with shiatsu treatments. When she has symptoms now, they are relieved through yoga.

She is entering menopause. Her last menses was in November 1992 (six months ago). Before this, her menses were regular and normal. For the past several months she has been getting an increasing amount of hot flashes, alternating too hot and too cold, and feeling more unstable emotionally. She feels depressed and experiences deeply anxious sensations in her belly from time to time. After a month or more of night sweats and sleeplessness, she started taking an herbal menopause formula that has helped control the hot flashes somewhat.

She stopped drinking alcohol two months ago. Before this, she had two to three glasses of wine every night in order to relax.

She has used marijuana intermittently over the years, especially to stimulate late-night work sessions.

"I get all excited about a dream. It is an excitement as if I'm intoxicated by the possibility, thinking 'this is the way I should go.' I want to drop everything and go that way, make a plan and move toward the new big thing. But I finally saw that these dreams didn't really fit with the reality of my situation."

"For 20 years I was either studying for, beginning practice in, or being a political activist in the development of my profession, working very long hours with little time off. I took the practice for granted while doing the big important political work." (She has done a great deal of political work for her professional association over the years.)

"I am 50 years old and I still haven't created my practice as I want it to be." (Cries.)

"In the late 1960s I felt a sense of hopelessness. Then I discovered chiropractic, and this became my hope. I became politically involved, because I wanted to make a contribution to something bigger than myself. I had a grandiose idea of saving the world with alternative medicine."

"It is easier to devote myself to a group, to be a visionary, to do what is needed. Big and important things, useful things, relating to a community outside myself. Meeting a real need. It is a lot harder to develop my personal practice, which seems small, not so compelling, and not essential, involving only my own self-interest."

"I love to work hard, to feel useful."

"It is very important to have a dream. I want to live and be my dream, but I'm not sure what it is, exactly."

She is in a new relationship and engaged to be married.

"I want a dream to unfold for us together. My constant working has been a cover for my difficulty with intimacy with men. In my relationships with men I have been dominated by a negative 'masculine' side of myself—perfectionistic, competitive, and defensive."

She grew up on the East Coast. "As a girl I was a tomboy, out in the woods, climbing trees, catching guppies."

"When I was 12, I was depressed. My father, who was a well-known public figure in the state, went to jail for several months for tax evasion. I was told about it only on the day he actually went to prison. I had no warning. I spent the summer just hanging out with the dog in the backyard. My mother 'handled' it. She just worked. We never talked about it. Then, when my father came home, she fell apart and was hospitalized for a while."

"Around that time I remember giving my lunch box to a needy girl."

"When I was 14, I wanted to save the world. I had an intense desire to find out how to do something useful."

"All my life I have been philosophically oriented, with a longing for a spiritual life."

"My energy is boundless, positive, optimistic. Anything is possible."

She has a tendency to stay up very late at night—reading, writing, thinking (2).

She likes to do several things at once.

Desires garlic (2), sweets (1), chocolate (1), and eggs (1).

Averse to sauerkraut (2).

She generally is not thirsty (1); prefers warm drinks (1) recently.

Her sleep is good, except for the hot flashes and a tendency to have active, busy, creative thoughts at night. Sleeps on her right side. Salivates every night (2).

As a child she had a recurrent dream. Two men in black cloaks would grab her girlfriend and cut her with long sabers. She had other scary dreams. She used to tell God she wanted a scary dream. She would pick one out of an imaginary file cabinet and hold it up to God. This was her way of tricking God, because she knew He wouldn't give her what she wanted.

For many years she did not have sex; not many relationships. She and her fiancé will live together this fall.

She has arthritis in her left great toe.

She has a long history of cramps in the soles of her feet and toes when she is tired, when her feet are in cold water, or during and after sexual intercourse.

> *King: We would like you to consider the two cases as one. What do you observe, what strikes you about the cases, and, in particular, what are the common elements?*
>
> *Afia Menke: They both have issues about saving the world, especially starving children. They are both politically active. What is going on outside is different from what is going on inside. They emulate their mothers' physical ailments. They both work at 110 percent. They are better late at night. They have issues around bearing children. They have scary dreams at night. They have difficulty with intimacy, and they are both critical and judgmental. They are averse to sauerkraut.*
>
> *King: That is a good list.*
>
> *Bob Ullman: They both had an incredible desire to be useful. That was repeated over and over in various ways. They have to be useful, and that leads them to overwork. They completely overwork themselves. They do several things at once. The need to be useful is really the center of each case.*
>
> *Jonathan Shore: You presented a lot of information, so it is hard to crystallize it. They are both extremely industrious. It seems to go beyond being useful. Both have the desire to do great things. One is climbing up high, and they both*

want to be important in some way. Also, there is a certain sensitivity. They both are actually quite sensitive, in a certain way, to the world around them. It isn't exactly sympathy. So, I came to a remedy from that. It is the homeopathic preparation of cocaine.

Marcia Neiswander: What I found so interesting was the metaphoric nature of the tree climbing and the rock climbing. It seemed to be a metaphor for their whole life pattern, of wanting to get higher, to pull up, to give more, to be more, to achieve more.

King: Do you think they share a feeling that causes them to want to "climb"?

Marcia Neiswander: Yes.

King: How would you describe that?

Marcia Neiswander: Without seeing them, it is hard to describe. My best guess would be that maybe there is a strong need to be acceptable. "If I contribute more, I will be okay. I will be acceptable. If I don't do enough, then I am not going to be okay. I have to contribute more in order to be an okay human being." Something like that.

Guy Kokelenberg: I noted the censoriousness and the industriousness, but I have a hunch that you included the salivation at night as well.

Helene Schwartzenberger: I get the feeling that the industriousness is covering up an inability to have a relationship with oneself and with the world as a human being, as an elemental person. In the first case, her not really wanting to have a child is, in essence, her rejection of her own "inner child" and herself as a person. This industriousness and this great desire to be great and useful in the world are really a cover for a sense of inadequacy and inability.

King: So, if you felt that way, what words would you use to describe that?

Helene Schwartzenberger: It is insecurity, loss of basic self-esteem, inadequacy, perhaps helplessness.

Murray Feldman: I think there is one other common element, a spiritual aspect. Even more than being useful, they are both looking for a deep existential meaning to life because their lives feel empty and hopeless.

King: Yes. There is the sense that the individual life is meaningless.

Liam McClintock: I agree that the key elements in the two cases are the usefulness and the industriousness. Boericke also agrees. He lists both these elements under the mental section of one particular remedy in his materia medica. In fact, these are the only symptoms he lists for that remedy.

King: And we will come to that remedy in a moment.

Elements in Common Between the Two Cases

We looked at these two cases and came up with a list of common elements:

- The individual life feels meaningless, hopeless, mundane, and trivial.
- Needs to be doing something useful and important on a global or large scale.
- Does several things at once.
- Independent.
- Judgmental.
- High energy.
- Works very hard.
- Productive and creative at night, with increased mental energy.
- Politically active.
- An element of climbing, going up.
- Red cheeks.
- Aversion to sauerkraut.

Analysis of Case Number 1
(Dr. Kipnis)

I won't take you through a long, involved process of analyzing the case because it is really much more simple than that. One could look at it superficially and prescribe Sepia, Nux vomica, or Sulphur. While it is possible for a polycrest remedy to have an unusual presentation, I think most experienced practitioners will acknowledge that they usually know when they are seeing something that is unusual or that they haven't seen before. Even if you don't know what it is, you usually know that it is not familiar. This was the feeling I had with this patient.

I believe the most important symptom in the case is the central feeling that her life is meaningless or purposeless. She feels a lack of peace. She is paralyzed. There is an image of a cave (fears caves), of being trapped down low in the dark. And there is the compensation for that, that she must work intensely, "110 percent," on something big and important to make her life useful and meaningful. She wants to leap up and do, to run and climb, or she will end up back in the cave.

The repertory does not really have good rubrics to describe this. Ennui, perhaps, is the closest we could come to the central feeling. And the compensation for this ennui is her industriousness. Along with this I added the rubrics, Useful, desire to be; Climb, desire to; and Exertion, physical, ameliorates. These, I believe, are really the essential elements in the case.

Figures 1 and 2 show what the analysis looks like, both with and without an emphasis on the small remedies.

It is a repertorization that is either really great or really useless. Most of the rubrics are very small, and no remedy strongly covers all of the symptoms.

In truth, I didn't do all this before prescribing. I am behind the times. I don't have a computer on my desk! I was very struck by what I believed to be the core of her case.

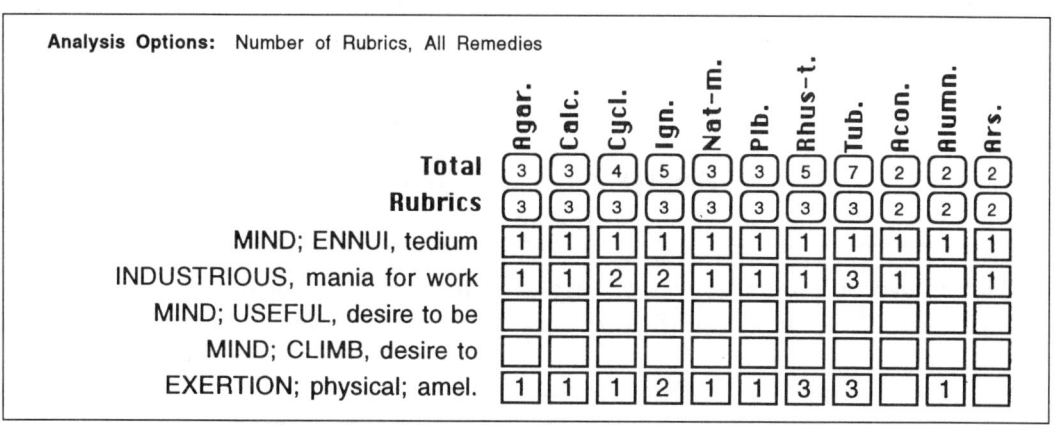

Analysis Options: Number of Rubrics, All Remedies

	Agar.	Calc.	Cycl.	Ign.	Nat-m.	Plb.	Rhus-t.	Tub.	Acon.	Alumn.	Ars.
Total	3	3	4	5	3	3	5	7	2	2	2
Rubrics	3	3	3	3	3	3	3	3	2	2	2
MIND; ENNUI, tedium	1	1	1	1	1	1	1	1	1	1	1
INDUSTRIOUS, mania for work	1	1	2	2	1	1	1	3	1		1
MIND; USEFUL, desire to be											
MIND; CLIMB, desire to											
EXERTION; physical; amel.	1	1	1	2	1	1	3	3		1	

Figure 1
Repertorization of the Essential Elements (Case Number 1)

237

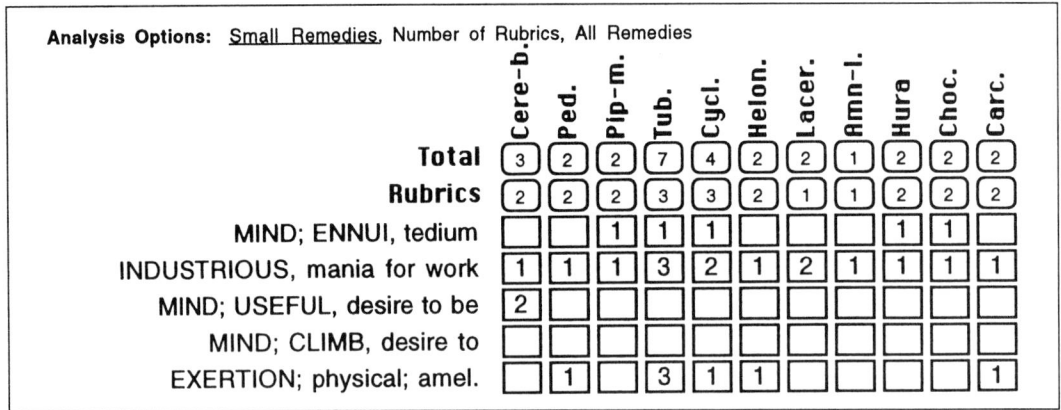

Analysis Options: Small Remedies, Number of Rubrics, All Remedies

	Cere-b.	Ped.	Pip-m.	Tub.	Cycl.	Helon.	Lacer.	Amn-l.	Hura	Choc.	Carc.
Total	3	2	2	7	4	2	2	1	2	2	2
Rubrics	2	2	2	3	3	2	1	1	2	2	2
MIND; ENNUI, tedium			1	1	1				1	1	
INDUSTRIOUS, mania for work	1	1	1	3	2	1	2	1	1	1	1
MIND; USEFUL, desire to be	2										
MIND; CLIMB, desire to											
EXERTION; physical; amel.		1		3	1	1					1

Figure 2
Emphasis on Small Remedies (Case Number 1)

So I thumbed through the repertory trying to find a way to get at this core. As I looked at the rubric, Industrious, reading each of the remedies and thinking about them in the context of the case, I came upon one remedy that I didn't know anything about. Curiosity took me first to Boericke and then to Allen to look for more information. In Boericke I found, "Great desire to work and to be doing something useful." In Allen it said, "Desire to engage at work. Desire to have the time all employed. Felt all day an astonishing inclination to be engaged in something useful."

I tried to find other confirmatory symptoms. It makes me uneasy to prescribe a remedy on essentially one symptom. But I couldn't find any others. There really wasn't anything else of great import. Everything that really bothered her emanated from the core and was compensation for it.

Analysis of Case Number 2
(Dr. King)

Her lower abdomen expresses stress in the form of constipation, a nervous stomach, diarrhea, hemorrhoids, and vaginitis. I find two main elements in this stress.

The first element is a mental excitement or intoxication, expressing itself in overwork and a need to do something useful and big—something important for others in the community outside herself. She wants to save the world. She has big ideas, searching for a dream that will provide the meaning in life. This is her stance in the world, her way of being in the world. What is this a compensation for?

The second element is an underlying sense of emotional hopelessness, smallness, unimportance, and self-doubt.

Converting these two elements to rubrics:

- Industrious.
- Fancies, exaltation of.
- Plans, making many.
- Useful, desire to be.
- Despair.
- Confidence, want of self.
- Delusion, smaller, sensation of being.

I repertorized both for all remedies and with an emphasis on small remedies (Figures 3 and 4).

Calcarea carbonica lacks good confirmatory symptoms but, more importantly, the essential issue of seeking protection or security (described well by Sankaran in *The Substance of Homeopathy*) is not really present.

Analysis Options: Number of Rubrics, All Remedies	Calc.	Chin.	Hydrog.	Nux-v.	Op.	Sulph.	Acon.	Agar.	Ambr.	Anac.	Ang.
Total	7	8	6	5	7	9	6	5	8	8	5
Rubrics	5	5	5	5	5	5	4	4	4	4	4
DELUSIONS; smaller; sensation of being	1		1					1	1	1	
MIND; CONFIDENCE; want of self	1	2	1	1	1	1			3	3	1
MIND; DESPAIR	3	1	1	1	1	3	2	1	2	2	
MIND; FANCIES; exaltation of	1	2		1	2	2	2	2	2	2	2
MIND; USEFUL, desire to be											
MIND; PLANS; making many		2	1	1	1	2				1	1
MIND; INDUSTRIOUS, mania for work	1	1	2	1	2	1	1	1			1

Figure 3
Repertorization of the Essential Elements (Case Number 2)

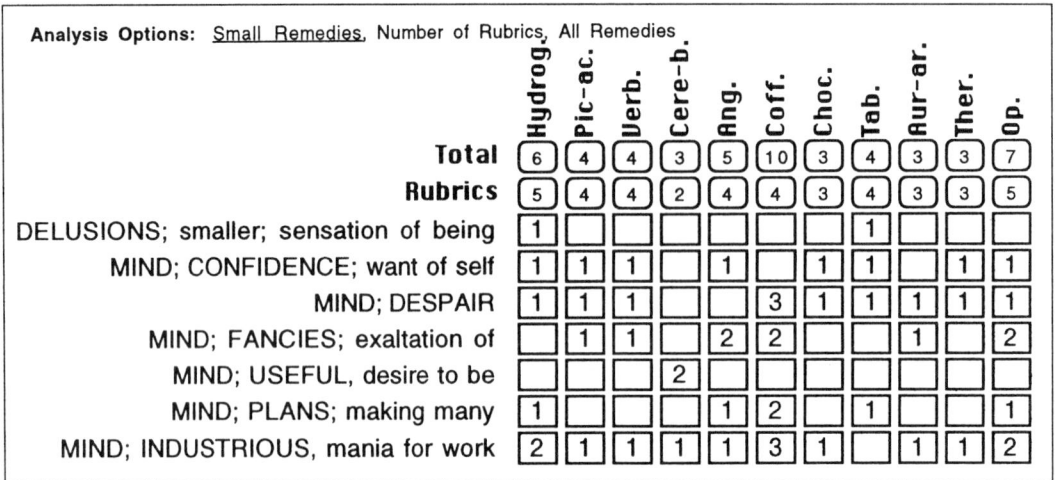

Analysis Options: Small Remedies, Number of Rubrics, All Remedies

	Hydrog.	Pic-ac.	Verb.	Cere-b.	Ang.	Coff.	Choc.	Tab.	Aur-ar.	Ther.	Op.
Total	6	4	4	3	5	10	3	4	3	3	7
Rubrics	5	4	4	2	4	4	3	4	3	3	5
DELUSIONS; smaller; sensation of being	1							1			
MIND; CONFIDENCE; want of self	1	1	1		1		1	1		1	1
MIND; DESPAIR	1	1	1			3	1	1	1	1	1
MIND; FANCIES; exaltation of		1	1		2	2			1		2
MIND; USEFUL, desire to be				2							
MIND; PLANS; making many	1					1	2		1		1
MIND; INDUSTRIOUS, mania for work	2	1	1	1	1	3	1		1	1	2

Figure 4
Emphasis on Small Remedies (Case Number 2)

I strongly considered China initially, but the case was lacking China's internal sensation of persecution—the delusion of being obstructed by others. And the China quality of dreaming big dreams but not really accomplishing much did not fit either. This is a woman who has accomplished a great deal.

I did not consider Hydrogen or Chocolate. The original repertorization was done with an earlier version of the Complete Repertory, which did not have the additions for Hydrogen or Chocolate.

Nux vomica certainly was a possibility because of the constipation, the other rectal symptoms, and the workaholism. However, my experience with people who benefit from Nux vomica is that their drive to accomplish is more "personal" or "selfish." They want to be the best, to win. It's a more direct form of egotism. This woman's drive is to accomplish something for the group outside of herself.

I also considered Cannabis indica, even though it does not come up as strongly in the repertorization, because of the big ideas, the grandiosity, and the mental excitement. But, as Ananda Zaren has described in her materia medica (*Core Elements of the Materia Medica of the Mind, Volume 1*), Cannabis indica has a pervasive element of dissociation—dissociation of the mind from the emotions and the body, and of the inner self from the outer world. This woman does not have this, nor does she have the hazy, out-of-control mental profusion I have observed in some Cannabis indica patients.

These considerations caused me to continue to look for a better prescription.

The Remedy Is Revealed

Cereus bonplandii is the remedy given in each of these cases. The need to have every minute of every day filled with doing something useful and important is the essence of these cases, and this appears to be the core of Cereus bonplandii.

Cereus bonplandii appears in the repertory very few times, from less than 20 times in Kent's original repertory to about 80 times, depending on which contemporary edition you look at. In comparison, Sulphur appears more than 15,000 times. (See Figure 5, the results of a MacRepertory/Complete Repertory search of the entire repertory—a total of 79 rubrics in which Cereus bonplandii appears.)

---

1. MIND; BUSINESS, desire for
2. MIND; BUSY
3. MIND; DEEDS, desire to perform, useful
4. MIND; DELUSIONS, incubus, being weighed down by
5. MIND; DELUSIONS, influence, is under a powerful
6. MIND; DELUSIONS, offended people, that he has
7. MIND; DELUSIONS, time, passes too, slowly
8. MIND; DREAMS, assemblies, large
9. MIND; DREAMS, dogs
10. MIND; DREAMS, events, long past, forgotten
11. MIND; DREAMS, fracas, of a
12. MIND; DREAMS, lewd, lascivious, voluptuous
13. MIND; DREAMS, noise
14. MIND; DREAMS, people, of, assembled
15. MIND; DREAMS, repeating
16. MIND; DULLNESS, sluggishness, difficulty of thinking and comprehending, morning
17. MIND; GENEROUS, too much

continues on next page

Figure 5
All Rubrics in Which Cereus Bonplandii Appears (Complete Repertory)

Figure 5, *cont'd*

18. MIND; IMPULSIVE
19. MIND; INDOLENCE, aversion to work
20. MIND; INDUSTRIOUS, mania for work
21. MIND; INSANITY, madness
22. MIND; INSANITY, madness, alternating with, physical symptoms
23. MIND; IRRITABILITY
24. MIND; LOATHING, life, of, menses, before
25. MIND; MENTAL SYMPTOMS alternating with, physical
26. MIND; MISTAKES, makes, time, in
27. MIND; PRAYING
28. MIND; RESTLESSNESS, nervousness
29. MIND; SIGHING
30. MIND; THOUGHTS, disordered
31. MIND; TIME, passes too slowly, appears longer
32. MIND; TRANQUILLITY, serenity, calmness
33. MIND; USEFUL, desire to be
34. VERTIGO; RISING, kneeling, from
35. HEAD PAIN; LOCALIZATION, Forehead, eyes, above
36. EYE; PAIN, General
37. EYE; PAIN, General, rising, when
38. EYE; PAIN, aching
39. EYE; PAIN, pressing, pressure
40. EYE; PHOTOPHOBIA
41. THROAT; MUCUS
42. ABDOMEN; PAIN, cramping, griping
43. ABDOMEN; PAIN, sore
44. MALE; ERECTIONS, troublesome, seldom, opposite sex, when with
45. MALE; PAIN
46. MALE; PAIN, Testes
47. MALE; SEXUAL desire, increased, night
48. RESPIRATION; SIGHING
49. CHEST; ANGINA pectoris
50. CHEST; EXPAND, as if expanded
51. CHEST; HYPERTROPHY of, Heart
52. CHEST; OPPRESSION, Heart
53. CHEST; PAIN, General, Heart
54. CHEST; PAIN, cutting, Heart
55. CHEST; PAIN, stitching, Heart

continues on next page

Figure 5, *cont'd*

---

56. CHEST; PAIN, tearing, Heart, region of
57. CHEST; TRANSFIXED, Heart, as if
58. BACK; ERUPTIONS, Dorsal region, Scapula, left, below, herpes like, with
    itching
59. BACK; ITCHING, Dorsal region, scapulae, left; below
60. BACK; WEAKNESS, Lumbar region, riding
61. EXTREMITIES; ITCHING, Knee
62. EXTREMITIES; ITCHING, Knee; bend of, right
63. EXTREMITIES; NUMBNESS, Upper Limbs, writing, while
64. EXTREMITY PAIN; GENERAL, neuralgic
65. EXTREMITY PAIN; UPPER LIMBS, writing, while
66. SLEEP; SLEEPINESS
67. SLEEP; SLEEPLESSNESS
68. SLEEP; YAWNING
69. SKIN; ERUPTIONS, eczema
70. SKIN; ITCHING
71. GENERALITIES; CLOTHING, intolerance of
72. GENERALITIES; CONVULSIVE movements
73. GENERALITIES; EMACIATION
74. GENERALITIES; FAINTNESS, fainting, rising, on
75. GENERALITIES; FOOD and drinks, dissolved food, desires
76. GENERALITIES; FOOD and drinks, sweets, desires
77. GENERALITIES; TRANQUILLITY, general, physical
78. GENERALITIES; WEAKNESS, enervation
79. GENERALITIES; WEAKNESS, enervation, riding, from
80. RELATIONSHIPS; Anhalonium lewinii, Lophophora williamsii, Peyotl, Mescal

---

Looking back at Case Number 2, we also see the confirmatory symptom for Cereus bonplandii of pain in the left side of the neck, a symptom that came out in the proving and is described in Allen. By the way, there is only one proving of Cereus bonplandii and it was done by only one person, a Dr. John Fitch.

Cereus bonplandii is a variety of night-blooming cactus that grows 30 to 50 feet tall. It is in the same family as the saguaro cactus, which grows very tall and straight up. It is a strong and vigorous plant. It is used for grafting other stocks and therefore is very "useful," giving up its energy for others. This cactus is an essential plant in the life of the desert, providing home and nourishment to birds, animals, and other forms of life.

It is interesting to note that both patients described having increased mental energy and productivity at night, "blooming at night." In both cases there is an element of climbing, of moving upward. And, in both cases and in the proving, there is a lack of thirst.

Follow-Up on Case Number 1
(Dr. Kipnis)

She was given one dose of Cereus bonplandii 200c on December 17, 1992.

January 27, 1993

She felt a tangible shift the day after taking the remedy. Things were rosier, and she felt more cheerful. She really felt the remedy made a difference, "like a weight had been lifted—calm, peaceful."

"The most pleasant feeling. Very profound."

She drew a doodle while talking on the telephone. It was very pretty and it served as a reminder of what she can do when she is not worried about what she's not doing.

Takes pleasure in the simple and mundane tasks of home and childcare.

Felt a flooding sensation of warmth along her left front leg several times.

Two days after she took the remedy she started to get a cold. Felt stuffed up. One week later she felt it was turning into a sinus infection. Because she was leaving soon for vacation she started using a decongestant and antihistamines. By the next day the feeling of well-being that she had for a week went away. The next couple of days she felt she was plummeting. She got so depressed she drank some coffee.

Six weeks after she took the remedy she reported that she did not regain the euphoric feeling she had right after taking the remedy. However, while she is still struggling, it is not as intense as before. For example, she is able to get up in the morning more easily.

She is not as nasty to people around her, although she is not much interested in them.

Has recently returned from a two-week vacation.

Her concern about the importance of what she is doing is on hold right now. She is considering going back into advocacy work. She feels she is taking action and therefore is not feeling frustrated or dissatisfied.

She hasn't had time to be depressed, bored, or disillusioned.

Assessment: Possible curative response.

Plan: Wait.

March 8, 1993

One week after the last visit she came down with another cold, with a sore throat, congestion, sneezing, and feeling achy. No fever and no sinus or head pain. She was sleeping well. She recovered easily with moderate vitamin support (vitamin C and beta carotene) and moist heat packs on the sinus areas.

She still goes up and down. But the highs are better—stronger and more even—and the lows are not as low.

Last week she felt listless; complete ennui. "I can't figure out what to do with the rest of the day. It stretches on, and I can't figure out how to get through it."

Since the last office visit she has had times where she has taken a real interest in exactly what's happening at the moment. Has moments of doing something mundane and enjoying it profoundly!

In the past she often did not get pleasure from what she was doing because she was rushing to try to produce something. Now she is more able to be in the moment and enjoy what she is doing.

The feeling seems fleeting, however. "I don't want it to slip away. It keeps me from feeling frenetic. I can't recall feeling this way since college." (Tears.)

"It has raised '10' to a new level."

She has lived with the feeling that every minute of her life had to be reflective of something, interesting enough for her to not be bored or depressed. Recently, for brief moments the struggle to make every five minutes important wasn't there.

She can get depressed from the self-consciousness of it all.

Her energy level is the same.

Her temper is definitely better. Situations that would normally set her off are not doing so.

She is sleeping okay. She is a little less sluggish in the morning on waking. Thinks to herself, "What am I going to get up for?" It's not as bad as it used to be.

Her sinuses are fine. The cold lasted only a few days. On the second day the congestion and pressure suddenly broke up and resolved.

Assessment: It always makes me nervous when a patient has an immediate and fantastically positive response to a remedy, and then crashes soon after. I needed to know how to best help this woman, and I could do this only by finding a way to distinguish between placebo response and response to the remedy.

Plan: Saccharum lactis (placebo), single dose.

April 26, 1993

She is doing okay but feels she is back to where she started.

She feels the last dose of the remedy did nothing.

When she looks back on the last 20 years she likes what she sees. It's the here and now that keeps her from peace. She is unable to just enjoy the moment.

She internalizes a lot because she works at home. She's not interacting with others. She second-guesses everything she does.

"Obnoxiously self-absorbed."

Since the first dose of the remedy she hasn't sunk to the depths of depression that she had before the remedy. "And I hope I'm not just saying that to make you feel good. I'm a very good girl."

(She says she believes she really hasn't been depressed.)

Assessment: The remedy action has been considerably weakened by the use of antihistamines and decongestants shortly after the first dose was given, resulting in a progressive relapse back to the original state.

Plan: Cereus bonplandii 200c, single dose.

June 3, 1993

Generally things seem more clear.

There is a decrease of the internal dialogue. Not such a muddle.

For weeks she has had a warm flooding sensation around the back of her left ankle.

No PMS or rage before menses the last couple of cycles.

Doesn't feel as frantic.

Her mother visited for one week. "I can sometimes be contentious with her, but I wasn't. I was in a better place to receive her. I was not as judgmental as I have been in the past."

Less anxiety. More willingness to let things happen. "This is something I was hoping to get out of all this."

She almost canceled this appointment because she was feeling so good.

She can run all sorts of internal dialogues but is able to short-circuit them, or they stop on their own because she is feeling more clear.

Appreciates all the positive aspects about her home and work situations.

Not feeling the need to push her career. "I've stopped pushing the river!"

Her decisions are settling in clearly and peacefully.

Her sleep is generally great. Still sluggish in the morning. Very slow to wake. A resistance to face the day, partly physical and partly psychological.

She had a realization two days ago: "If you feel you have to control the whole day, it's a real burden."

Assessment: Curative response to the remedy.

Plan: Wait.

November 10, 1993

She felt really well, with steady improvement, until two weeks ago.

"The internal dialogue made me completely dissatisfied with what I do. So much existential chatter. Eventually I got really depressed, wondering if what I was doing was really important."

She had a big upset over her work. Her boss didn't call her for several weeks despite her requests. She took it personally and felt unworthy and downtrodden (2). All the same feelings that her internal chatter is about. Felt an immediate flood of relief when her boss finally called.

Got sick a week later with headaches and then a relapse of her general condition.

Assessment: Possible relapse.

Plan: Wait one to two weeks to see if patient rebounds on her own.

(On November 23 the patient called to say that she was no better, and the remedy was then repeated. Cereus bonplandii 200c, single dose.)

February 11, 1994

Telephone consultation.

She has had an intermittent headache for the past month. Has generally ignored it. This week the pain is in her ears.

A week ago she started hurting behind her ears, especially on the left. It is low-grade, constant, dull, and itching. Earlier in the week it radiated to the occiput. It slowly subsides when she is sleeping at night. It returns within one or two hours of being upright. Feels better with covers up around her ears. No discharge from the ears. No fever. She never had anything like this before.

Her energy is normal.

Assessment: Acute viral illness.

Plan: 1. Vitamin C, 500 mg three times a day.
2. Beta carotene, 25,000 IU twice a day.
3. Moist heat packs applied to involved areas twice a day.

April 25, 1994

Telephone consultation.

She is feeling good. Definite progress has been made.

She felt she had "fallen off" last autumn. "It was a good experience to know what it felt like to have problems again and then have them resolved."

Occasionally she has flashes of the rage and feeling of insignificance. "The things that used to bother me so much just aren't present!"

"It's really very clear to me that there is a difference over this long period of time."

"Things are pretty even now."

No problems with sinuses for a year or more.

Her inner ear problem resolved within one week after the last telephone call.

"I will never forget the time after I first took the remedy. The reaction was so dramatic. I had an interest in drawing and in ironing tablecloths. I felt a newfound joy in really basic activities."

"The high doesn't exist now, but it served its purpose. It helped me to see the lows. It is very clear to me that something very dramatic has been happening."

Assessment: Continues to improve.

Plan: Wait.

Follow-Up on Case Number 2
(Dr. King)

The initial dose of Cereus bonplandii 200c was given on May 5, 1993. Here is a brief overview of the follow-ups, followed by the complete information:

Two doses of the remedy, both 200c, eight months apart.

An episode of yeast vaginitis soon after the first dose and then nothing other than an occasional sense of irritation.

Slow and gradual improvement in the constipation, resulting in normal function. Intermittent hemorrhoids.

Cessation of the hot flashes for seven to eight months, then a milder return of symptoms, and then cessation again.

Normal menstrual period (May 1, 1994), unexpected, one year after the initial consultation. No menses since.

Persistent increase in the upper back and neck tension and pain; worse on the left side.

Significant reduction in anxiety and feelings of uselessness or worthlessness; increased ability to live in the present in a relaxed manner despite considerable stress in recent months, especially around the sickness and death of her father.

Increased ability to pursue an intimate relationship with a man; not escaping into work.

No more tendency to mental excitement and making grandiose plans late at night ("night-blooming").

July 13, 1993

She is doing very well.

The day she took the remedy she had yellowish diarrhea. That evening she started to have vaginal yeast symptoms—itching in the vulva and vagina—that persisted for a few days and then went away. No further yeast symptoms.

The day after she took the remedy she had an easy and complete stool, and then the stools became more frequent as they had been previously. But her stools are hard and incomplete most of the time (2).

The hot flashes went away completely for six weeks and then returned in a different form. They are not as intense; heat moves upward from the upper torso; they last about one minute; and they occur every few days. She is no longer taking any herbs to control the hot flashes.

One month after she took the remedy she had a very slight menses, one drop of blood and a small amount of mucus.

Soon after she took the remedy she had a painful, purple, protruding hemorrhoid, with slight bleeding of bright red blood. It lasted for one month and then went away. She had her first hemorrhoid at age 13; it was associated with constipation.

Soon after she took the remedy she stayed up late, until 2 a.m., with high energy and excitement. Making plans.

Her fiancé is going to move in with her in two weeks. She is looking forward to this.

She is investigating various possibilities for improving her practice, such as new locations and setups. But she has not been feeling that things must be absolutely perfect. She has a more relaxed feeling about it.

She has had some right lower back pain, but it is not bad. No left neck pain.

Occasionally she gets a "nervy" tingling sensation in the right ischial tuberosity. Used to get this before menses.

Assessment: Improvement.

Plan: Wait.

September 21, 1993

No hot flashes, only a rare brief warm feeling.

No yeast vaginitis.

Her bowels have improved. She has the sense of incompletion with the stool less often. She does not need to be as rigorous with her diet to moderate the constipation. When she is nervous, she may have a hard stool with gas.

One month ago, for a while, she had an old symptom of brownish, thick, gelatinous postnasal discharge in the morning. (Usually gets this at this time of year?)

Recently she has had shooting pains in the left temple and inside the left ear. Long history of this happening occasionally.

Two weeks ago, for a short time, she felt useless. She was wondering what would organize all her interests. But basically she has felt well.

She is now living with her fiancé. It's going well, wonderful. Not feeling a need to run from the relationship as she might have in the past. Sometimes the relationship is hard for her. She gets scared that it won't really work, that there won't be a real "union."

Her sleep has been good. Not having the high energy at night. Not needing to stay up late.

She has had a few cups of coffee, and some marijuana.

Assessment: The improvement is continuing, despite some potential interferences (coffee and marijuana).

Plan: 1. Wait.
        2. Stress importance of avoiding coffee and marijuana.

December 7, 1993

She is doing remarkably well, especially considering recent stresses and changes:

Just found out her father has metastatic cancer.

Her mother had a recent colonoscopy because of blood in the stool.

She moved her office to a new (and better) location.

She and her fiancé moved to a new house.

"In spite of all this, I am feeling basically well. I'm not becoming deeply anxious about things, as I would have in the past. This remedy has helped me to be okay in the present."

Still no hot flashes. It is now over a year since her last normal menses.

Her low back went out from lifting during all the moving, but the discomfort wasn't bad. Then she got a cold with a persistent hard cough, and the cough aggravated her back. The back problem was relieved after she had some adjustments.

Two or three weeks ago, she felt as if her pelvic area "flashed" or "flared." Pain in the right ischial tuberosity extending to the right labia. She had a hemorrhoid, probably associated with some constipation at that time, and she had some vaginal irritation. All of this subsided without treatment. No symptoms in the past one to two weeks.

Her stools have been normal most of the time. During the pelvic "flare-up," she had experienced some sensations of rectal insecurity, which she had previously. Once, she lost a small amount of brown liquid during flatus.

The night before she heard about her father's cancer, she dreamt that there was a grape-like cluster or growth inside of her that broke off in her hand. In the dream the feeling was of surprise, not alarm.

She feels positive about her relationship. She feels committed. Sometimes it is difficult trying to communicate. "I want tenderness and empathy from my fiancé, yet I don't give this to myself. To be kinder to myself means knowing that what I am doing right here and now is okay, without needing my previous role as a leader in my profession in order to feel okay. Giving up all of that was like a loss." (A few tears.)

She has not been staying up late.

Used some marijuana during the recent moves.

Assessment: The improvement is continuing, but perhaps slowing because of stress of father's health problems.

Plan: Wait.

December 31, 1993

Telephone consultation.

She thinks she may need to take the remedy again.

Ten days ago she had some bouts with constipation. Hard, pellet-like stools. This ended four days ago with some diarrhea.

"It's probably related to emotional upheaval and stress. My family has been around for the holidays. My sister says I act like the Queen of Sheba, uppity. A part of me is like this, and another part feels clumsy, like an adolescent boy. I am more aware of these two aspects than I was in the past—a feeling of confidence and a feeling of boyish clumsiness. I am giving myself more credit for my own power in the work I do in my practice."

No hot flashes.

Used marijuana once.

Assessment: A possible partial relapse.

Plan: 1. Wait.

2. Send one dose of Cereus bonplandii 200c, to take if she continues to feel a decrease in her general state over the next ten days.

February 8, 1994

She took the dose of the remedy on January 18, 1994, because she began having hot flashes ten days before. Also, there was more constipation with pellet-like stools, some left neck pain, and several days of the same useless, negative feeling she had experienced previously.

After she took the remedy her bowels and neck were immediately better. Then, after a while, the symptoms returned. She has been constipated on and off. The left neck pain has been bad again recently.

The hot flashes did not change after she took the remedy. But the pattern is somewhat different. They occur mostly while she is in bed at night or in the morning on waking at the normal time (6 to 7 a.m.). They are mild and do not last long. And she does not have the emotional instability that she had originally.

New symptom: Her eyeballs feel dry, especially on waking in the morning.

She has a hollow pain inside her left ear, associated with a tender left occiput, and a deep pain in the left upper back.

Despite the stress of her father's illness ("slowly dying") and the stress of her fiancé's inability to find a job, she generally feels much better mentally and emotionally. "So much better. I am less defensive, more relaxed. Things are easier. Despite the stress, I feel that things will be okay."

She is going to the Caribbean for a week vacation in mid-February. "I need a little time away."

Assessment: It is too soon after the second dose to evaluate the case thoroughly, although some positive effect is apparent. Overall, the patient is doing well.

Plan: Wait.

March 23, 1994

Telephone consultation.

Her father died at the end of February. "I don't feel unfinished about it at all. A lot of love was expressed."

She had some constipation during vacation, and developed acute diarrhea on the plane ride coming back. She took one dose of Veratrum album 30c and was better. Since then her stools have been softer and more regular. No pellet-like stools, and she feels more in touch with a normal urge to pass the stool. Sometimes she still has a sensation of incompletion, but it is less intense than before.

She has had three dreams involving stools.

Has used marijuana occasionally.

Assessment: Continues to do well.

Plan: Wait.

April 4, 1994

"I'm doing pretty well."

She is doing quite well physically.

No hard stools. Regular, softer stools in the morning. No feeling of incompletion. Recently some discomfort from hemorrhoids, with a bit of bright red blood.

"My abdomen doesn't feel as dead or numb as it used to."

Her hot flashes are calming down. Most nights she has a brief hot flash around 4:30 a.m.

Feels tight and stiff in her back (1).

Recently she had left neck pain, shooting upward to the left side of her head. "Inside the head." Had some bodywork done on her neck.

"I miss my father, but I am okay. I felt very conscious through it all. It was a good experience. My mother is having a hard time. I feel torn between being here with my fiancé, who wants more attention from me, and being there with my mother." (Cries.)

Assessment: Stable state, with continuation of increase in musculoskeletal symptoms.

Plan: Wait.

May 23, 1994

On May 1 she had a normal menses, which lasted five days. Very unexpected!

Her stools were normal until just before the menses, then she was constipated for two to three days (usual premenstrual pattern for her). Stools were normal again after this. Then recently she had a few days of constipation, associated with some stress in her relationship.

Also her nipples were sore before the menses, as with her menses in the past.

"The whole thing seems to be about my difficulty in having an intimate relationship. At times I am very critical of him. He still hasn't found a job. I become impatient with his 'victim' tendencies. And my mother needs my help. I should be there. I feel tension about this. Then I feel uncertain about staying in the relationship. I seem to pick out men who are 'wounded.' My first husband was that way, too."

"I'm only beginning to understand how central my father's going to prison may have been in my life. It was a public shame for him. My mother just worked, never talked about it. I always felt sorry for my father. I felt my mother nagged him."

Her left upper back and neck are gradually worsening; chronically stiff and tight.

Clenches her teeth at night during sleep.

Her low back has not been a problem.

She drinks one cup of coffee most days, for the past month.

Used marijuana once.

Assessment: The improvement is holding, and she has more insight into herself.

Plan: 1. Wait.
2. Stress importance of avoiding coffee and marijuana.

Description of Another Case
(Dr. King)

I have another patient who has responded very well to Cereus bonplandii. The follow-up period is only six months, so I will describe only the general elements of the case.

She is a 36-year-old "high-energy" office manager in a busy sales and marketing firm. I began treating her in the spring of 1992. In the past she had spent many hours doing volunteer work for various organizations.

Her original complaints were a tension in the left hip ever since a sports injury five years before, a tendency to low back pain since adolescence, persistent fatigue (mother of two young children), and an inability to take good care of herself in terms of eating right and exercising. She also had occasional sinusitis with green nasal discharge since a bad flu at age 22.

I had given her several remedies without significant benefit, including Sulphur, Calcarea carbonica, Veratrum album, Arsenicum album, Phosphorus, Ignatia, and Belladonna.

She has red cheeks (as in the other two cases). She speaks loudly and forcefully, leaning forward. Here are some quotes from various visits:

> I am a positive person. I have an inherent inability to allow myself to be depressed. I just go and do things—clean out the closets, make a list. People don't want to hear a sob story. I tell them things are great. I have very little patience for being bummed out or feeling self-pity. It's hard to be sympathetic with depressed people. I am sympathetic only to a certain point.

> I am very active. I rarely do only one thing at a time. I will sew, pay bills, fold clothes, and watch a video movie rental all at once.

> I am a logistical thinker, a practical thinker. I think of potential problems that might arise. I focus on the details. Things are planned into the future.

> When people say it can't be done, I just push harder and work harder. I work very fast and very hard, like an adrenaline rush. I press myself to meet my goals and deadlines. I set a bigger goal so that I will reach the realistic goal. It's not external forces that make me go so fast. It's me.

> So many things to do simultaneously. No time. One thing after another. Things hang over my head. Hurried. I am behind. I am on overload.

I can be very self-righteous and judgmental. I am quick to think I am right, to know the truth. I can react quickly and get angry, but I don't argue with people. When people have a difference of opinion with me about politics, religion, or other things I can write them off.

People say I am an extrovert. I am very expressive and sensitive—easy to laugh, blush, cry—but I like my privacy. As a child I was a "space cadet," frequently staring out the window. Even now I often day-dream, imagining future scenarios and redoing past events with different outcomes. (This is a proving symptom: Re-dreamed old dreams in part or whole.)

I have positive memories of my childhood. I was naive and protected, always felt special. A good, well-behaved girl, even as a teenager.

My mental state depends on how well I juggle everything. Can I pull it off? I go from one activity to another. My self-worth relates to what I have accomplished that day. What I do is what I am. Without this I become less focused and kind of depressed. It is hard to let things just be the way they are.

I have never liked intense intimacy. I didn't want anyone to be that needy with me. It would be suffocating. When I was 15, a boyfriend dumped me. I never told anyone or showed what I felt, just sat and stared out the window.

I have the feeling that I can't let my guard down for a minute or I will get behind. There are a lot of things I want to do in the world. I have a lot to offer. I have a need for community. There is so much to be done. I want to learn more and be valuable to my company. I want to be used up by the time I die.

This woman reported an increase of energy in the evening, when she would work on projects. She also had a strong aversion to sauerkraut. It gives her headaches. (This aversion was elicited after the remedy was given with benefit.)

The patient has thus far had one dose of Cereus bonplandii 200c (January 1994).

After the remedy she reported the following:

> I feel freed up from all the "have to's." I used to think I had to be frantic in order to be productive and useful. Now I can let things be slower and quieter. And I still feel productive. I can turn things over to others to do. Things fall into place now. I am making time for little pleasures for myself. I am a lot more centered, not as interested in being "good," doing what I ought to do. I can let myself be "bad." I have needs that may conflict with others' needs. I have put a lot of things off for many years. I don't have to do everything for everyone else and always accommodate others.

She had not responded to any of the previous remedies in this way. She has also done very well physically.

Looking again at the elements in common between the first two cases, we can see that this third case shares many of these: a high energy level; a red face; a very active person who works very hard and does several things at once; an increase in mental energy at night; a judgmental nature; and a strong need to be productive and useful.

In this case, however, there does not appear to be the element of climbing. Also, the focus of this woman's life is less global. She is more focused on family and home, although she is very dedicated to her company.

Symptoms from the Proving Confirmed by These Cases

Following is a list of symptoms from the Cereus bonplandii proving that were also present in one or more of the three cases. The numbers after the proving symptoms indicate Case Number 1, 2, or 3.

Mind

- Desire to engage at work. Desire to have the time all employed. Felt all day an astonishing inclination to be engaged in something useful (1,2,3).

- Experienced an agreeably tranquil frame of mind and body (1).

- Arose feeling miserable (1).

- Very irritable (1).
- Very dull all morning; passed the time in a listless manner. Time passed very slowly (1).
- Felt a desire to give something quite necessary to myself to another (2).

Head

- Pain verging around and along left parietal bone from left occiput (2).

Ear

- Pain behind mastoid process, left side, extending backward and upward (1,2).

Nose

- Accumulation of mucus in both nostrils. Mucus from nose, as in catarrh (1,3).
- Greenish discharges from right nares; similar discharge in less quantity from the left (3—recurrent sinusitis with green nasal discharge).

Stomach/Abdomen

- Relish for sweet things (2).
- Thirstless (1,2).
- Griping pain in epigastrium (1).

Stool

- Copious and urgent evacuation from the bowels (2).
- Stool not easy nor sufficient (2).
- Effort to evacuate bowels nearly or quite ineffectual (2).

Neck and Back

- Pain on left side of neck (2).

General Symptoms

- Each night seemed to be under the influence of something powerful (2).

- Do not know what to do with myself (1).

Sleep

- Late at night, but not sleepy (2).

- Re-dreamed old dreams in part or whole (3—in her daydreaming).

Roger van Zandvoort: This element of wanting to go up, the climbing upward, is exactly what this kind of cactus does. The saguaro cactus, the candelabra cactus, is in the same family. Many of the cacti in this family don't even have side branches. They have one nucleus that goes straight up into the sky. There are different kinds. Actually, Cactus grandiflorus is a Cereus, too, in the same family. It probably has a similar mental quality to Cereus, although we don't know that.

Also, these two patients were thirstless, and cacti are desert remedies. Maybe it is no wonder that Cereus is a thirstless remedy.

Sharon Ryals-Tamm: I don't have any experience with the remedy. I do, however, have a question. When we give a remedy like this to "pathological" activists, does it make them less effective in the world? They are very useful, you know. (audience laughter)

Kipnis: Well, I can speak only from this one case that I have seen. She is still politically involved and still productive, but without the "pathological" drive and the angst that was driving it. She still has the desire to do something useful and productive in society, but it is no longer a "pathological" need and she is not suffering from depression along with that need.

Steven Olsen ND, DHANP

A CASE
OF
PARANOID
SCHIZOPHRENIA

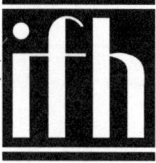

Steven Olsen is a graduate of Bastyr College of Naturopathic Medicine and for the past six years has been in private practice in Coquitlam, British Columbia. Steve has taught homeopathy at both Bastyr College and the Ontario College of Naturopathic Medicine. He also teaches acute and first-aid homeopathy in his community. Steve regularly has attended George Vithoulkas' seminars in Germany and elsewhere over the past several years.

[Editors' Note: Before beginning his formal presentation, Dr. Olsen took the audience through a guided meditation involving music and visualization. The music was expansive, at times bombastic. The images invoked were those of unity—moving beyond normal boundaries of identity to a oneness with the universe, a universal truth. "You are a microcosm of the universe, a tapestry of all that has existed before. You are a living consciousness. You are an expression of many elements, energies working in harmony and balance.... Imagine yourself walking toward the center of your own being. There you find a unity, a oneness, the center of your own creativity. There you find the possibility of all things...you break the boundary...you have touched the invisible...." Dr. Olsen's comments made while presenting the case are bracketed and italicized.]

Introduction

When I was about 14 years old I had a type of existential crisis. I told my parents this whole western world we lived in was "totally useless." I begged them to send me to India or Tibet. There I would be taught to meditate, I would reach a higher state of consciousness, and then I would be free and find total happiness again. They said they wouldn't send me. I wept in despair and then said, "Well, I may as well stay here and make the best of it." What was the element within me that had such a yearning?

This is a case of a 45-year-old man who was treated successfully for paranoid schizophrenia. His main symptoms were delusions of persecution, paranoid ideas, delusions of grandeur, thought disorder, flaws of reasoning, and auditory hallucinations. The only treatment he received was two doses of homeopathically prepared Hydrogen.

The idea for this prescription came from the proving done by Jeremy Sherr, RS Hom. I am sincerely grateful for the very excellent work he has done. The text of the proving states:

> In the beginning was hydrogen.... It was the first element to be formed in the universe.... Being the first, it is a link with "the time that was before" (a phrase from the Kalahari Bushman). It is the "first born element" being both positive and negative and possessing pattern, or structure. It is also the most abundant element in the universe. (*The Proving of Hydrogen*, Jeremy Sherr, The Society of Homeopaths, Artizan Road, Northampton NN1 4HU, England.)

Hydrogen is also the source of all things. Every other element is made of this basic unit. It is the unity of all things. It makes all things possible. It is the source. It is the beginning of energy and matter.

Was there an energy or consciousness that brought this first element into being, or is this energy the great creator itself? Can this element still have a memory of this event or of its creator, or how did it create itself? Does it know itself, know all the other elements it has been infused into, know all other molecules in the universe, know all living things, know human consciousness so it now can ponder itself and continue on its mission? Is it therefore the essence of "life" itself? Does it know what it wants from us and where it is going? It seems to be very creative, creating more and more complex forms of life. It has a big ego to take on such a task.

There are literally billions of hydrogen atoms in each person. What role does it play in the developmental process? Does it try to impress its "will" on us to return to the source of all things—a higher state of being, back to divinity—to complete its goal? What happens when this element becomes too powerful within us, what symptoms are created, and how does the balance become restored so that the healthy development of the person can once again continue?

This case is the story of a man's journey into the unknown. He describes it as "an important mission with global implications." He spent many hours, weeks, and months in meditation, reading esoteric literature and thinking about how to make positive and creative solutions in his life and the lives of others. Then there was a breakthrough. His mind made a connection with a supreme life force. Here he found eternal truths, revelations, and experienced excitement about the possibilities before him. Just as in *The Allegory of the Cave* by Plato, it is the most difficult of tasks to have a revelation, to see "another reality," and then to come back and try to explain it to people who see only the "shadows on the wall."

Along the path to complete his mission something went wrong. His perception became distorted, the information did not integrate into the real world, the ego became too inflated, and past unresolved conflicts came to the surface. Eventually, the state of higher consciousness became too much to handle. It is at this point that I had the opportunity to work with him and help him to find a way back.

I hope that I have given credit where it is due, minimized errors, and maintained respect and dignity for the patient who gave me permission to present his very personal story.

Initial Visit: August 27, 1993

Male
Age 45

Observation: My first impression is that this patient has an intensity about him. His eyes are staring at me in a super-concentrated manner. His movements are fast and precise. His nervous system is on the alert. He is very awake.

His first words to me are, "Steve, you are on level four."

Then he pauses as if some great revelation has just entered his mind. "I am on level six. I know we are going to be able to work together, Steve. I can't tell you everything right now because it is complicated and you will soon understand when you are ready."

[*From this brief interaction I could already choose some rubrics:*

- *MIND, Haughty.*
- *MIND, Egotism.*
- *MIND, Theorizing.*
- *MIND, Abstract.*]

"I am on a mission to put together a spiritual army. I met a spiritual guide, but it is more abstract than that. It is the source of all things, a oneness. The universe wants the oneness. Now I can sense the answers to questions. It is as if I know everything. I know 73 languages now. The universe is speaking through me, like a God but not religious. A type of mind with a purpose to achieve the best. I also believe that I have superhuman strength."

Then he asked me if I would let him hold my hand so that he could teach me homeopathy. I said, "Sure, go ahead." Then he took my hand lightly and proceeded to "transmit to me all the homeopathic knowledge" that he had made contact with. His eyes were turned upward and he blinked rapidly as he performed this procedure.

[*I came up with some more rubrics:*

- *MIND, Delusions, absurd, ludicrous.*
- *MIND, Delusions, greatness of, as to.*
- *MIND, Delusions, enlarged.*
- *MIND, Delusions, God, that he is in communication with.*
- *MIND, Delusions, great person, is.*
- *MIND, Delusions, knowledge, thought he possessed infinite.*
- *MIND, Delusions, superhuman, is.*

Hydrogen is a new remedy, so it did not appear in any of the rubrics in my repertory. But if the symptoms I mentioned are repertorized you can get an idea of the remedies that can be compared with Hydrogen.

Using the Synthesis Repertory of RADAR, Sulphur appeared in first place, followed by these remedies: Platinum, Veratrum album, Lycopodium, Lachesis, Nux vomica, Silica, Stramonium, Cannabis indica, Arnica, Aurum, Mercurius, Paris quadrifolia, Hyoscyamus, Alumina, Opium, Phosphorus, Pulsatilla, Conium, Sabadilla, Palladium, Calcarea carbonica, Staphysagria, and others.

It is interesting how many of these remedies have aspects to them of "expansion." This is in contrast to remedies like Cyclamen, Natrum muriaticum, and those in the Baryta or Cuprum family that are all very contracted, cramping, and introverted. Out of these expansive remedies we need to find one that fits the other aspects of the case.]

Repeats words (2). "I have to repeat things three times to keep a balance. I call these "triples."

He used to be organized; wanted people on time (1). Was a perfectionist (2).

"I was a workaholic in the past, but now I don't have a regular job. I will sit for hours staring" (2).

He was artistic and creative in the past; did some acting (1).

He read a lot for a year. Was "swallowing" books on religious and philosophical subjects (2).

Will go into a trance if you don't talk to him (2).

Speaks in idioms for balance (2).

Has fixed ideas, such as "Dairy is not good" (2). Connects to ideas on the essence level of things (2).

Has extreme health beliefs (2).

Last year he was into dowsing with a pendulum (2), then didn't need it anymore (2). "The universe is fine-tuning me."

He has problems communicating with people (2). Swears, curses, uses gross, ugly, sexual words (2).

Low self-confidence (2).

Never cruel.

Fears? None.

He cried when his wife left him.

No conflict with sexual feelings.

Takes control of a group (1). Wants to lead (2). Dictatorial (2).

"We will have a team (2). I am knowing the answers."

Some paranoia. "Someone is trying to kill us." Won't let his girlfriend walk past the window because he is sure someone will shoot her (2). Tackles her if she walks past the window.

"Spirit is all" (2).

Talks of travel (3). Wants to travel to meet up with other people who will help in the mission (2).

"I want to let the spirit take over" (1).

Delusion: "My father went to jail for molesting kids" (2).

[*This is a delusion. This did not happen. The rest of the family was in the room when I took his case. His girlfriend, his son, his parents, and his brothers were all there to help and support him. I don't know if he wanted them there.*]

>   **Audience:** *Did he know they were there?*

>   **Olsen:** *I think so. His girlfriend was crying intermittently as we went through it.*

Oneness of everything (2). "The universe wants the oneness" (2). "The universe is talking through me" (2).

Wants to achieve the best (2).

"It is all one" (2).

[*As I am taking the case I feel as if he is floating away. I need to find something to bring him back to earth. What could have caused this? What is he unable to face in reality to have made the choice to leave his body in such an extreme way? Is he bored with reality, is it grief, is it the ego trying to take total control?*]

He married when he was 19 years old. He has two children (1).

Divorced his first wife and then got married again. The second marriage lasted eight years.

Since his last divorce he has been on a spiritual quest (2). Science of Mind church. Owned a construction company and then sold it. Quit the church. "Then got more into my trip." Used to be athletic but not in the last two years (1).

Has never abused drugs or alcohol (2).

Physical symptoms:

- Warm.
- Shaky.
- Dry mouth and lips.
- Tight stomach.
- Eyes move rapidly when he thinks (2).

In the last two years he has been sleeping only one to two hours each night (2). Problems sleeping through the night (2).

Eats mostly vegetables and fruit (2). Also red meat, kiwi, and raisins.

Quite thirsty (3). Craves warm, room temperature, or hot drinks (3).

More sensitive to cold (1).

Olsen: What are your impressions?

Audience: Grandiosity, delusion.

Audience: Did he feel that there was something wrong, that he needed treatment?

Olsen: He did want to get better. In later follow-ups we will find out more about this. In the paranoid state, he would tell his girlfriend, "I feel sick. Take me to the hospital. I know I am sick. Something has gone terribly wrong with me. I need help. I believe in what I am doing but something has gone wrong."

Christopher Jayne: How long has he been in this state?

Olsen: He has been in this more severe paranoid state for three or four weeks, and that is when he really started to get worried. Before that, he wasn't worried.

Marcia Neiswander: His sleep is unusual. It is characteristic of psychotic behavior. What is the cause for all this?

Olsen: I was trying to find some kind of etiology, but I had a difficult time discovering one. The only etiology I could find was that he really was searching for spiritual enlightenment and truth for many years. It seems that he learned and developed and was creative in that endeavor, but something did go wrong.

Sheryl Kipnis: I am still confused about how long he has been in this state.

Olsen: Well, for at least two years he has been moving more and more into his own belief system, becoming more and more carried away with these ideas. The intensely paranoid ideas, I believe, have only been around for about a month. Some of the stranger ideas about what he knows, the delusions of grandeur and so on, have been much worse in the last month, to the point where he is uncomfortable with it.

Sheryl Kipnis: Was there pathology prior to the past month?

Olsen: No. He undoubtedly had a lot of ideas about things, but you would probably have described him as "eccentric" rather than psychotic or delusional.

Analysis: An Unwilling Traveler into the "Twilight Zone"

This patient made a definite impression on me. First of all, he had only a few physical symptoms. I felt that his consciousness had expanded to the outer limits of the universe and had found something there. It is an experience, perhaps, that many people are trying to achieve—transcendence from the physical boundaries and into the mystical spiritual realms. In a sense we all want to "take off from this planet" and go back to our original "home" where there is a oneness of all things, before we differentiated into individual beings. To become an individual is often a grueling and painful process as we face loneliness, selfishness, and alienation from meaning. To find the way back requires the development of many qualities from within. Disease is there to keep us on this path.

In this case I believe the desire to develop the capacity to unite with the "source of all things" was premature and led to a certain type of imbalance, distortion, and breakdown. As one author puts it, "The road to enlightenment is littered with the wrecks of souls that were not ready for the powerful forces that are generated from such action." (*The Gateway to Liberation* by Mary Gray.)

This patient is in a diseased state because he no longer has any choice over his thoughts and actions. His perceptions have taken control, and he has increasingly become the unwilling traveler into the "twilight zone." Also, many of his experiences can be classified as absurd claims, excitable fantasies, and paranoid delusions.

There is still a question as to what is real or true in his experience and what is fantasy, imagination, and delusion. I would consider the following as real: the realization that we are all connected, the conviction that we need to help each other and the planet if we are to survive and continue to develop, the intuition or inspiration that we can bring new ideas into positive action, and the experience of ecstasy that comes with a spiritual experience.

We are now in a position to add to the repertorization already in progress:

- MIND, Absorbed, buried in thought.
- MIND, Abstract.
- MIND, Anger, from contradiction.
- MIND, Audacity.
- MIND, Boaster.
- MIND, Clairvoyance.
- MIND, Confusion, identity, as to his.
- MIND, Contradiction, intolerant of.
- MIND, Cursing.
- MIND, Deeds, great sensation as if he could do.
- MIND, Delusions, conspiracies.
- MIND, Delusions, injury, is about to receive.
- MIND, Delusions, enemy, surrounded by.
- MIND, Delusions, pursued, thought he was.
- MIND, Delusions, voices, hears.
- MIND, Ecstasy.
- MIND, Excitement, excitable.
- MIND, Exhilaration.
- MIND, Expansive.
- MIND, Fanaticism.
- MIND, Fancies, exaltation of.
- MIND, Fearless.
- MIND, Foolish behavior.

- MIND, Impetuous.
- MIND, Impulse, peculiar.
- MIND, Indolence, aversion to work.
- MIND, Insanity.
- MIND, Introspection.
- MIND, Mania.
- MIND, Meditation.
- MIND, Optimistic.
- MIND, Passionate.
- MIND, Plans, making many.
- MIND, Prophesying.
- MIND, Religious affections.
- MIND, Schizophrenia.
- MIND, Schizophrenia, paranoid.
- MIND, Selflessness.
- MIND, Sits, wrapped in deep thoughts.
- MIND, Slander, disposition to.
- MIND, Speech, foolish.
- MIND, Strange things, impulse to do.
- MIND, Suspicious.
- MIND, Sympathetic.
- MIND, Travel, desire to.
- MIND, Theorizing.
- MIND, Thoughts, profound.
- MIND, Thoughts, rush.
- MIND, Withdrawal from reality.
- SLEEP, Waking often.
- STOMACH, Thirst for large quantities.

I used RADAR and the Vithoulkas Expert System to repertorize, which resulted in the following remedies: Sulphur, Stramonium, Lachesis, Hyoscyamus, Aurum, Veratrum album, Ignatia, Cannabis indica, Anhalonium, Opium, Nux vomica, and Belladonna.

Although there are aspects of these remedies that fit this case, there is none that fits better than Hydrogen.

Plan: Order the remedy Hydrogen.

Durr Elmore: Using MacRepertory (with the latest edition of the Complete Repertory, which has additions for Hydrogen), with an emphasis on the small remedies, the analysis of the rubrics you chose for the case yields Anhalonium (peyote), Androctonos (scorpion), and Cannabis indica. The sixth remedy that comes through the analysis is Hydrogen.

Olsen: I'm sure that it will come through with the additions from the proving.

Follow-Up

September 1, 1993

(Remedy not yet taken.)

He wants to go to Los Angeles today. No matter what I say he insists on going. He says he is going to meet a team of people, and they will make plans to do some great deeds. He has no idea who these people will be. (I am convinced he will go to Los Angeles, meet someone else in the same state of mind, and then end up in India—never to be heard from again.)

Assessment: Paranoid schizophrenia.

Plan: Hydrogen 200c, single dose.

September 15, 1993

Observation: His eyes are more restful. The movements are not so agitated.

He just got back from a trip to Los Angeles, New York, and Edmonton.

[Editors' Note: The next several comments are in the patient's own words.]

Overall, I feel better. My mind is calmer. I have come back.

I went through some erratic stuff a while ago. I know I dragged my family through this. It was necessary.

It didn't feel okay for me to be so way out and weird. It was a hallucination based on my emotions not working or on negative emotions.

I am more integrated now, back into my physical body (2).

I was doing things that were abnormal during the three-week period when things went haywire just before I came to see you.

I wanted to get close to the invisible and unite with it (2).

I had to deal with pollution, people being sick who I wanted to help, the state of human thinking (1).

On February 5, 1993, I felt some bodily discomfort, which lasted until recently (1), such as sore muscles (2), twitching, various sensations running through my body (2).

Before I took the remedy I had communications in the back of my head. I heard voices (2). This has stopped now. One voice bothered me. It was a very critical voice that exposed my family or said things that were not true, sexual things (2). Now I feel these voices were there to assist me in a cleansing process. It made me accuse my father of sexual abuse. It was going on 24 hours a day (1).

I know now this was not true. I wanted to experience what sexuality was so I could help people that were sexually abused.

The voice is no longer negative (1).

It was very scary and unpleasant to be in that state.

His girlfriend says, "He is back to his normal, old self. Before he came to see you, he had a bad period of 3½ weeks. I had decided to leave him and not see him anymore." Then four days later he started to leave his body and he said he loved her (2). The next day he had to be taken to the emergency room. It was as if he was in shock (2): dry mouth (1), chills (2), blank look (2).

"In the hospital, I (girlfriend) said to him, 'Look at me.' He said 'I hate you' and 'I am dying.' I prayed for him and took him out of the hospital because the doctors wanted to give drugs to him. Then we left together, looked in the telephone book, and found you—the naturopath."

He was afraid that if he and his girlfriend became too involved he would feel trapped. "I want to be free." He wouldn't commit to her. But he also was afraid that he could not live without her. She wanted to end the casual relationship because he would not make a commitment. Then he flipped out (2).

Then he kept walking in a daze and having hallucinations (2). He said to his girlfriend: "Mary, talk to me. There are cops outside the door." He kept wanting to be taken to the hospital. "There are guns pointed at us." Wanted to go to the airport. This was out of character for him (2), according to the girlfriend. She then called his parents. "I moved him to my place. The next day we brought him (2) to see you. Now, we are friends again" (2).

He says, "I will look for my own place to live now. It is sad I can't give her what she wants." (More of a relationship; more intimacy.)

He is not as thirsty now (2). He was drinking two quarts a day.

He is tired from all the traveling, being away for 11 days (1).

He is taking some vitamins.

He eats only vegetables, chicken, and fruit (1).

He began to receive information from non-physical communications about a year ago. He took notes on it and read a lot (1).

Assessment: His ego is back under control (2). He is not expanding into the universe anymore. The remedy is correct.

Plan: 1. Wait.
       2. Return in one month.

October 5, 1993

(Video excerpts were shown.)

He was in New York for a while. Wore the same clothes for a week.

Drives around in his car all day (2).

Is somewhat in denial (1).

He is obsessive about perfection (2).

Contradictions are unacceptable for him (1).

Reclusive (2).

Says he can know things telepathically (2).

He is talking about traveling again, to California (2).

He presents an image of having lots of money (1).

Still feels he has special powers (1).

Rationalizes (2).

He wants to save the world (2). Big plans (2).

In a fantasy world (2). Big ego (2), but low self-worth (2). Pretends he has control (1), but inside he is a baby (1).

No paranoia.

Goal: employment (1).

"I am receiving cosmic information every day (1). Universally directed (2). Ideas from the universe (2). I am growing from them to assist the planet, wellness, pollution." (2)

Wants to go to Los Angeles today (3).

Abundance of self-confidence. (2)

Assessment: Relapsing. I need to see him improve within 48 hours or refer him to a psychiatrist.

Plan: Hydrogen 200c, single dose.

November 10, 1993

In general, he feels better again.

No physical symptoms (1). Some tooth pains (1). More physically active; walking more (2).

Abstract mind (2).

He is learning about the process (1), the future (2), the work (2). Gaining insights (1).

Goal: trying to get insight into it. It has to do with addressing the negativity on the planet—sickness, people becoming aware (2).

"I can't share it all with you. It is the invisible, non-physical aspects of the universe. This is what I am concerned with. This is becoming more clear to me. The plan is very intricate, long range. To bring peace and quiet to this planet. It will take a number of years working with various people to accomplish it."

He is not reading now. Used to do a lot of reading. Now he rides around in a car, soaking up information (1). "I receive various ideas (1) that I don't understand but things are getting more clear." (1)

He is staying with his girlfriend, who has teenage girls.

Good moods. Good social contact with friends and family (1). Visits people (1). Talks on the telephone. Visits with his son. Enjoys seeing people (2).

"I still believe I will do lots of traveling" (1). Still has the desire to travel (2).

"I was off balance" (1).

"There is an answer (2). It has been kept from people on this planet (1). Something to do with oneness, synthesis" (2).

Struggles with the opposites of the universe (2)—individualization versus synthesis and the meaning of wholeness (2).

Assessment: Doing better.

Plan: Wait.

May 20, 1994

I talked with his girlfriend on the telephone.

He is a bit eccentric about his ideas, but basically he is doing okay.

He still does not have a job and isn't looking for one.

We both feel he is not totally better. But he is not paranoid, he is not traveling as much, and his moods are stable. He does not feel there is anything wrong with him and does not want another appointment at this time.

June 8, 1994

I telephoned him just before this conference. He doesn't feel a need for further treatment at this point.

"I am doing well, 100 percent better."

He has no paranoia. "I haven't had any symptoms that would require medication."

"My learning process continues. It will take a number of years. I still have insight, but I don't really want to explain it right now."

He enjoys visiting people and talking on the phone.

He is not reading now.

I spoke with his girlfriend. They still live together. She says he is fine.

He likes to travel and feels he will, but he doesn't have the desire to just take off anymore.

"I was off-balance before."

"I don't talk to anyone about my belief system anymore. Most days I feel relaxed and in a good mood."

(I asked him about religion.) "In any religion there is a spark of truth, but we aren't supposed to really get into it right now. We aren't supposed to become totally spiritual right now."

(I asked him about all the problems on the earth, all the conflict and war.) "There is a beingness that is in synchronicity. "Conflict is a necessary form of expression. It is a selfishness and a violence that people have to experience and that the people around the violence have to experience. The people around the violence are inspired more strongly for compassion. I am very optimistic about the world, and I understand why there has to be negativity and conflict."

Assessment: He is philosophical and matter-of-fact about his ideas, more modest.

Some Notes on Hydrogen

Hydrogen, like many other remedies, has a range to its therapeutic efficacy. So, although I have chosen the following symptoms from the proving to support this case, I do not want to present this information as a fixed essence of Hydrogen's "genius."

In Jeremy Sherr's proving of Hydrogen the following experiences were recorded. (The notation after each listing refers to the number of the prover, the potency taken, and the day on which the symptom was experienced. Thus, "16, 30c, 06" means the sixteenth prover, the thirtieth centesimal potency, on the sixth day. Where the day/time was irrelevant or unclear it was marked as "XX.")

> I feel I have moved into a different state of consciousness and there aren't any guideposts or means of navigation—a bit like being lost in space. 16, 30c, 06

> Feeling like visiting another dimension and having to come back here and it's all the same as it was before. 16, 30c, 08

> There is a very fine line at this time between enlightenment and insanity—a split consciousness. The dark side is horrendous, but the positive side of the proving has been well worth it. The positive aspects

are beautiful. It's a shame we need to come down. I guess the price of going to heaven is a trip to hell. 16, 30c, XX

I've experienced a lot more egotism in the last few weeks. I feel frustrated by the limitations of the ego. 16, 30c, XX

I feel so much love I don't know how to focus it. It's like being in another state of consciousness. No one can come near and it's frightening me. 16, 30c, 25

I felt the presence of a totally pure energy, like meeting God and feeling totally unworthy or like meeting a lover and feeling unworthy— realizing all the mistakes of a lifetime. This pure energy was around for some time protecting me. I feel this unification cleared out lifetimes of symptomatology for me.... I felt overflowing love for humanity and wanted to give everything away. My mind turned to Buddha. It was like seeing the complete picture instead of fragmented bits. (These primary effects lasted about 28 days, then changing to a paranoid state.) 16, 30c, 07

My whole time scale changed since taking the remedy. I've lost a lot of boundaries on time. Don't hurry, just do things in my own time. 08, 30c, 06

It seems as if all the days became one. 16, 30c, XX

I became silly and manic, rushing around. 24, 30c, 00

I feel distant and separated from things and they feel unreal. 16, 30c, 01

Fear that someone was trying to find out if I was home so that they could come and rape and murder me. 16, 30c, XX

Feel I can't trust anyone. Paranoia. 4, 30c, 100

While sitting in a restaurant, felt progressively more cut off from friends at the table. I began to feel detached and paranoid. I felt disliked by people. They seem to look at me menacingly.... I felt very uncomfortable and wanted to get out. I put my head down and rushed out saying good-bye, feeling a sense of relief at getting away (all very unusual for me). Outside, I felt relief and my mind cleared and I walked home alone. 22, 12c, 04

I think that no one likes me. I felt betrayed and everything went haywire. 16, 30c, XX

A spark of a paranoid thought. Maybe I'm being poisoned. 10, 200c, 00

Felt cut off from people and suspicious. 22, 12c, XX

Greatly increased tendency to theorize and philosophize, especially concerning esoteric matters. 16, 12c, 05

I didn't have the opportunity to read these proving symptoms until long after my patient had received the Hydrogen. I believe these proving symptoms confirm that he was given the correct medicine.

In reading the literature on schizophrenia and paranoid schizophrenia I was amazed at how many of these symptoms were covered by the remedy Hydrogen. It is especially interesting that schizophrenia can produce so many bizarre religious ideas and that mental hospitals have to keep religious ideas away from the patients because it makes them much worse. They have already progressed too far in that direction. Perhaps this is not a rare remedy for that condition.

There is a well-known affliction of a type of religious mania that ordinary people get when they visit holy places like Jerusalem. Hydrogen may be one of the medicines to treat it.

It often takes an extreme case to prescribe Hydrogen for the first time. Once we know the pattern of an extreme case we will be able to recognize the same pattern in more ordinary circumstances. The pattern of symptoms we can look for is as follows:

- Strong sense of self-confidence.

- Sometimes egotistical.

- Episodes of extreme excitability about spiritual things.

- Bright smile with eyes wide open, saying: "I have found the answer. I have really found it."

- Expansive.

- History of being very energetic.

- Paucity of physical symptoms.

- Theoretical, inspirational.

- Charismatic.

- Full of new ideas.

- Creative.

- Over-excitable, religious; "new age" extremism.

- Independent in thought but want to work with others.

- Sympathetic, working for a cause.

- Bored with the norm.

- Anger if contradicted.

- May feel alienated at times from other people, or alone in their quest, or sensitive to the fact that other people do not agree with them.

Most times we would incorrectly give Sulphur (egotism), Veratrum album (egotism, haughty, religious mania, bipolar moods), or Medorrhinum (egotism, expansive nature, excitability, delusions).

It is a tragedy that without homeopathy these people would end up in a mental hospital with various medications and very little chance of cure. This person did not have a support system in place to help him through his initiation process. Our society simply is not set up for these people. There needs to be a revolution in psychiatry so that these patients have the opportunity to choose homeopathic treatment. I am hopeful that one day we will see this become a reality.

Afia Menke: What did you feel when he was in the Hydrogen state. What kind of feelings came over you sitting in the room with him? Did you believe him? Did you feel kind of "taken in"?

Olsen: I have, of course, seen patients with big egos—people needing Sulphur, Veratrum album, Platina, and other such remedies; people who think they are superior and can do anything; people who put other people down—where the egos seem greatly "expanded." However, I felt that this man's ego had gone beyond the earth! It's unfortunate that the first interview was not videotaped so that you could see that.

Audience: You felt as if you went there with him?

Olsen: No. I didn't go there with him. Perhaps I could just feel through him where he was. It was incredibly expansive with an absolute kind of arrogance, as if he had found something and he was going to dictate it to everyone else. He wouldn't accept anyone else's ideas. Now, after the remedy, he is not so arrogant. He is not trying to force his ideas on anyone anymore. He is not "out there" like he was.

Marcia Neiswander: Sometimes, when you are with somebody who is quite psychotic, some of the things they say to you can ring true. Sometimes they say a lot of spiritual-sounding yet bizarre things that may come across as exactly correct, even though the person is totally "out there" in many other ways.

As I watched him on the follow-up video, I felt that he is still not "connected." He is still somewhere else. It is as if he is lecturing you from another place, like there is a part of him that is still very disconnected and that is spiritually somewhere else. The two still have to come together.

Olsen: I think it is accurate to say that he did go somewhere, and he truly did experience something that the average person doesn't experience. A part of him was healthy, I think, and I don't want to take that away from him. I feel that he is on a path and he is going to work it out. I don't feel that this is the end of the journey.

Richard Hiltner: Did he practice any formal meditation? And, secondly, where can you get the remedy Hydrogen?

Olsen: He did practice meditation. I don't know exactly what type. Both the Helios and Quinn pharmacies have the remedy now.

Richard Hiltner: Was the meditation done before, during, or after this psychotic episode?

Olsen: It was for one to two years beforehand.

Richard Hiltner: Did he have a guru?

Olsen: Not that I am aware of.

Nancy Herrick: There is a new classification for this kind of state. It is called "spiritual emergency," and you actually can fill out your insurance forms with this as a diagnosis. I think it is a better classification than paranoid schizophrenia.

Also, I thought it was interesting that many of the other remedies that came up for consideration were drug remedies. Yet he presented in a very "mineralized" kind of state, with his general appearance and even his striped shirt. He looked like a businessman.

Olsen: Yes, he looks very proper.

Helene Schwartzenberger: Many people who go on spiritual quests apparently go to mountainous areas. It is my understanding that it is not an uncommon phenomenon for spiritual crisis to happen in these settings in higher altitudes. I wonder if there is an excess of hydrogen in higher altitudes?

Eric Sommermann: There is somewhat more hydrogen in the higher atmosphere.

Sharon Ryals-Tamm: I know of four Hydrogen cases, one that I treated and then three others from colleagues. It is interesting that in each of those cases the patient had not used drugs or alcohol. They were very "clean." They were in this expanded state without any drugs. In one case the patient was a teenage boy whose father was sure his son must be using drugs because he was in such a hallucinogenic and psychotic state.

The person I treated had been a spiritual seeker all his life. He was the kind of person who didn't want his own name. He took a name from one of the many paths he had followed. The reason I treated him was not for the spiritual seeking, as such, but rather for his intense feeling of separation. This is what I saw in all four of these Hydrogen cases. It is not a minor sense of separation. It is an agony that is nearly incomprehensible to ordinary people. They don't feel like they belong to the human race or to the planet. The sense of being alone is massive. It is just beyond anything we can imagine, and the fear that comes from that is tremendous.

After taking one dose of the remedy my patient said nothing happened. However, he actually became very successful in the spiritual practice that he was involved in. He became a teacher and became a very gracious, humble person. Before the remedy, he knew it all but he was such an egomaniac that people couldn't stand to be around him. He also had no ability to just be with human beings in a natural way. He couldn't hold ordinary jobs. After the remedy, he got a good job with a computer company and women started chasing him! He is still a very spiritual person, but he is successful in expressing his spirituality in a very generous way, in a way that actually contributes to other people.

What I saw in those four Hydrogen cases is that people don't actually give up a spiritual quest. Rather, they are able to integrate the spirituality into their lives. They can bring in the light that they are seeking in a way that makes a difference on the planet.

Marcia Neiswander: *I'd like to make a short comment on schizophrenia. It is odd that this man developed his symptoms at that age. The normal onset of schizophrenia is in the early to mid 20s. As we learn more about Hydrogen, I wonder if we might discover that this remedy corresponds to psychotic problems that develop in the 40s as part of the psychotic element that occurs in the 40s with a spiritual midlife quest or crisis.*

Durr Elmore: *I had a very interesting Hydrogen case that is a little different from the one you just presented. This man was very sane and, in fact, I felt he was a very high spiritual person. He had had some experiences of enlightenment. This was a man with kind of a natural spirituality. There was no egotism. He wasn't connected with any particular movement or guru. As a child he had some ecstatic experiences. He said that when he was in his mid 30s he experienced a complete oneness with Buddhahood, with the universe. He was in this state of complete spiritual bliss for about three or four weeks, and then he gradually came down and had a difficult time integrating it into the world. He went into a kind of depression that lasted for about a year, at which point he was referred to me.*

I didn't feel a lot of pathology there, but I had heard Jeremy Sherr lecture on Hydrogen—about the up and the down of the remedy. This man was up with the oneness with God and then down into the quagmire of the world, not knowing what to do. So, I gave him one dose of Hydrogen 200c and the result was just beautiful. He integrated so well into the world. Before, he was meditating for hours a day and not able to function in the world. After, he took a job, became enthusiastic about it, and got married within six weeks! He has done very well since then. He still is spiritual, but it is very balanced. This is a remedy we have to consider for spiritual seekers, especially people who have been "high."

Barbara Dively: The end result after Hydrogen sounds something like the end result after near-death experiences, where there is a union with the oneness and they have a whole different view of religion and life, but yet it is positive. They come back and do not preach their message, yet they retain a different vision. Any comments on that?

Olsen: I think that is right. I think something very positive did happen to my patient, although there were difficulties. Some people probably take this path and are able to go more slowly, maybe have someone there to help them through it, and they do fine. They come back very humble people and integrate the experience into their lives. It has a very positive effect. I think it is only when there is a lot of conflict, when the ego gets too big or some such side effect, that we would have to give this remedy to help them through that crossroads.

Don Beans: I would like to say thanks for opening up my mind one more time, just as Roger Morrison and Nancy Herrick did in their seminar, "Metaphysics and Madness." They brought the question up several times: Where is the line between a metaphysical experience and insanity? I think that is something that we really need to pay attention to. I see in your presentation of this case that your feeling is not so much of madness but of a metaphysical experience. You have been really helpful in helping me to understand this.

Nancy Herrick: I would like to make the point that all people who are in this state are not Hydrogen and, specifically, that there is another very similar state expressed by the remedy Anhalonium.

Olsen: Have you had any experience with that remedy?

Nancy Herrick: Well, we have been discussing the differences here in the back of the room. The consensus seems to be that Anhalonium has more a sense of great love with a lot of visions and colors—much more of a sensual feeling and a merging with their surroundings. As I said before, I was struck by how matter-of-fact he appeared on the video.

Lawrence Vannekirk: I'd like to comment on what Barbara just said. If you look at Aphorism 215 in the Organon, Hahnemann talks of mental disease being the result of a suppressed corporeal disease. And, in 216, he goes on to say, "The cases are not rare in which so-called corporeal diseases that threaten to be fatal...become transformed into insanity, into a kind of melancholia or into mania...whereupon the corporeal symptoms lose all their danger and these latter symptoms improve almost to perfect health." So, I am wondering if there isn't actually a relationship, as you say, to a near-death experience?

Anne Schadde: When I was in India I saw a case of Anhalonium that was very interesting. It had the element of merging with the universe. The woman described how she sat at the seashore and had the feeling that she and the seashore were one. When she went to the ancient places where the old people lived 500,000 years ago she had the feeling as if the ancient time was still there. She was within the ancient time, and yet she still also lived in this century. She had become very sick one year before. She said, "I was lying in the bed, thinking that even when I die there is nothing wrong with me. I can never die in my life. Nobody ever dies."

This is a bit different from my understanding of Hydrogen, which is more disconnected from the world. Hydrogen is "outside," and the world is here. Anhalonium is perhaps more down to earth, and they have the feeling of merging together with everything, merging with the universe.

Audience: Anne, what were they trying to cure in the Anhalonium case?

Anne Schadde: She was very sick. She had pneumonia.

Barbara Newlon: Paul Herscu talked about an Anhalonium case that he cured. The woman presented with colitis symptomatology, very physical symptoms. She described an experience that occurred while sitting on a rock near water. It might have been the ocean. She felt a oneness, as if she could just merge with the water with no concern for her own survival. She then just slipped into the water. She would have drowned except that a man came by, saw her, and pulled her out of the water. She was, however, a person who had done a lot of drugs and this was a way of life for her.

Olsen: We haven't made the remedy from phencyclidine (PCP) yet, but the people who use it do very unusual things and their belief system is incredibly distorted. They do things like run up to the top of their apartment building and *just fly out onto the concrete. They must have some incredible belief about who they are and what they can do. I heard of a man who jumped from his apartment building, fell on a hedge, got up, ran back up to the top of the building, jumped again, and hit the concrete. We need to do a proving of that for people who have delusions of being able to fly.*

Guy Kokelenberg, MD,
and Roger van Zandvoort

COMPUTER-ASSISTED ANALYSIS IN DIFFICULT CASES

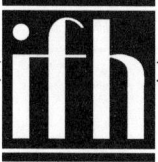

Guy Kokelenberg worked for six years as a general practitioner before encountering classical homeopathy through Dr. Bladys. Guy studied further with Dr. Imberechts at Homoeopathica Europa, where he later taught. With other homeopaths in Belgium, he founded the VSU, a school for classical homeopathy. He has had his own practice in Belgium for the past eight years and has worked for many years with Dr. Dockx on the Comparative Materia Medica.

Roger van Zandvoort is well known to all MacRepertory users around the world as the creator of the Complete Repertory. This is an expanded computer repertory (also coming out in print soon) that incorporates many thousands of new remedies, new rubrics, and additions to existing rubrics.

Introduction:
A Small Remedy Produces Constitutional Results
(Dr. Kokelenberg)

I just took 1 kilogram of Argentum nitricum, three Valiums, and two shots of whiskey. Now I feel reasonably calm and ready to speak (audience laughter). It is a good feeling to travel halfway around the world and realize we are working with the same books, using the same homeopathic language, and having the same ideas. It is like coming home to "family" again. It feels nice. This is my first time here. You will have to kick me out, because otherwise I will stay!

Before I begin my formal presentation, I'd like to tell you about a delightful case, one that taught me a lot. In my practice I have frequently treated a patient unsuccessfully for chronic problems until there is an acute illness that shows me the person's constitutional remedy. This case is an example of this phenomenon. I learned a great deal from this case.

The patient was a 70-year-old woman who came to see me several years ago, with a chief complaint of Ménière's disease. She had vertigo attacks every one or two days, sometimes more frequently. It was terrible for her. She no longer left her house to do things. She was anxious, afraid, and depressed. As a consequence of the disease, she had deafness and a constant ringing in the right ear. In addition, she had repetitive sore throats with formation of white offensive plugs on her tonsils, especially on the right tonsil.

I took her case for quite a long time. She was a very industrious woman and rather bossy, especially at home with her family. She gave a strong impression of being easily frightened when there was something wrong with her. She had suffered from infectious hepatitis with jaundice during her adolescence.

I gave her a dose of Lycopodium 200K (Korsakoff), and the frequency of the Ménière's attacks was reduced to every two weeks or so. She was considerably better. The sore throats were also less frequent, although they did not disappear completely. There were several follow-ups over more than a year, and no other remedy was given.

One day her daughter called to tell me that her mother hadn't slept for two weeks because of a pain in the back. Conventional treatment had been unsuccessful. No etiology could be found. The patient came in and described the pain. It was a stitching, burning, sharp pain, localized in a spot in the dorsal region below the right scapula. She couldn't lie on her right side, which was her normal sleeping position. The pain persisted day and night, a terrible pain.

Initially I felt confident because Chelidonium, which is complementary to Lycopodium, is well known for pain in this location. I thought that this was a Chelidonium case that I mistook for Lycopodium. The two remedies are similar, and this is why Lycopodium had an effect. This will be a quick consultation!

I was very close to writing a prescription for Chelidonium. However, when I considered other symptoms in her case that weren't completely cured—the recurrent sore throats and the plugs on her tonsils—then I wasn't so certain about the remedy. Chelidonium is not listed in the rubrics, THROAT, Hawks up cheesy lumps, or THROAT, Caseous deposits in tonsils.

In addition, I noticed something strange. Most people with deafness in the right ear will turn their left ear toward you in order to hear better. This woman, however, sat with her right ear turned toward me! This seemed very odd. When I asked her why she did that she said, "I can't stand the traffic noise." It was about six in the evening and there was a traffic jam outside my clinic. But, as I talked to her, she kept asking me to talk louder! I asked her if my talking louder would hurt her. She said, "When you talk loud it is okay. Otherwise, I don't understand you. But, if there is street noise, I can't stand it."

This was indeed strange. I looked in the repertory and was fortunate to find what I needed. She had impaired hearing for the human voice. In Kent's repertory (page 323) there is a rubric, HEARING, Impaired, voice, the human. Take a look at the remedies in this rubric and compare them with the remedies in the previous two throat rubrics. Also, look at the remedies listed under BACK, Pain, dorsal region, scapulae, right, under (page 902). Then go to HEARING, Acute, noises, to, sounds of vehicles, although deaf to voices (page 321). It was the sound of traffic she couldn't stand. Only one remedy is there. It is a remedy that is in each of the other rubrics—Chenopodium anthelminticum.

I didn't know the first thing about this remedy! I opened Boericke. What concerned me was that this woman's main pathology was the Ménière's disease. Back then, we used the rubric, EAR, Noises in, vertigo, for Ménière's disease. Chenopodium was not in that rubric, and that bothered me. I know we can give a remedy anyway, but I like it if the remedy is known to cover the patient's chief complaint. [Editors' Note: In the Complete Repertory, Chenopodium has been added to the above rubric, as well as to a new rubric for Ménière's disease in the Vertigo section.]

In Boericke, I found the following, which made me feel much more comfortable:

> Characteristic pain in scapula very marked.... Sudden vertigo. Ménière's disease. Affections of auditory nerves.... Ears—Torpor of auditory nerve. Hearing better for high-pitched sounds. Comparative deafness to sound of voice, but great sensitiveness to sound, as of passing vehicles and also a shrinking from low tones. Buzzing in ears. Enlargement of tonsils. Aural vertigo. Back—Intense pain between angle of right shoulder blade near spine, and through the chest....

I was happy to see that Boericke listed Chelidonium, which I had been considering, under remedy relationships for Chenopodium. So, I confidently prescribed Chenopodium anthelminticum 200K, one dose. She went to the pharmacist. He called me to ask if I had made a mistake, because he did not know the remedy and he most certainly did not have a 200K! This was on a Friday evening, and pharmacists in Belgium don't work on the weekend.

He searched around and found a 6K dose of Chenopodium in a drawer. That was all he had, so I told him to give it to her. I thought it would at least do something for the subscapular pain, even if it didn't do anything for her Ménière's syndrome. I instructed the patient to repeat the 6K three times a day.

On Monday she phoned me and said the pain in the back was immediately better after beginning the remedy. She was able to sleep from the first night on, and she didn't have any vertigo. The vertigo had been better with Lycopodium, so it was premature to evaluate the effect of the drug on the Ménière's.

I told her to discontinue the Chenopodium and wait. She came for a follow-up one month later and reported only one vertigo attack and no more sore throats. The tonsillar plugs and the deafness on the right side were still there. I then prescribed a dose of 30K, because I had the illusion that the deafness could also improve, which unfortunately was not the case.

Two months later she told me there had been no more vertigo attacks, no more sore throats, and no more tonsillar plugs. The pain in the back was definitely gone. Only the deafness in the right ear remained, which is still the case today. I see her frequently, because her grandchildren come to me and she accompanies them. Her family tells me she is also less bossy.

Lessons Learned from the Chenopodium Case

This case can teach us some important lessons:

- First, there are no small remedies. A remedy is called "small" because we don't know it or it hasn't been proven. A small remedy can act constitutionally.

- Second, we must continue to make additions to the repertory from materia medica so that we have the best possible chance of finding the correct remedy in each case.

- Third, we can frequently find the remedy a patient needs in an acute illness. It is therefore important that we organize our practices so that we can see our patients when they are acutely ill.

- Fourth, the potency is not important. The potency is absolutely irrelevant for me anymore. Even a few doses of a low potency can produce a deep constitutional result, as we saw in this case.

Before this case, I had two anxieties. I worried about finding the remedy, and I worried about selecting the "best" potency. Now, I have just one anxiety—finding the remedy (audience laughter)! I always give 200c and that works out fine.

An Aside: A Worm Is Expelled

Chenopodium is a vermifuge. Oil of Chenopodium kills worms, which reminds me of one of the first cases that convinced me of the efficacy of homeopathy. A boy in the neighborhood had been stammering for a long time. Nothing helped, not even antidepressants and a year of psychotherapy for the child and the family.

I decided to take his case. It looked to me like a Baryta carbonica case, but I wrote the prescription very small because I wasn't very confident (audience laughter). I gave a dose of Baryta carbonica 200K. This was also on a Friday, and I told his mother that if something happened I would be home the next day. I wasn't confident, you see.

The following morning I had some consultations and the mother came to the clinic. She brought a jar with her, the type you would use for marmalade. In the jar was a worm, a roundworm one meter long, that her son had evacuated the evening before! From that moment on, he never stammered again. Can you imagine?

I could not find an allopathic connection between worms and stammering until this year, when it was mentioned in one of the journals that someone had observed a connection. Baryta carbonica is not listed in the repertory for stammering, so I added it, in pencil.

Roger van Zandvoort: Baryta carbonica has been added for stammering in the Complete Repertory. The source is Boenninghausen. I don't know whether he knew about the worms, but he knew about Baryta carbonica and stammering.

Kokelenberg: I will erase the pencil and put it in bold now (audience laughter)!

Roger van Zandvoort: In the first degree, I would suggest.

[Editors' Note: We have bracketed and italicized Dr. Kokelenberg's spontaneous comments. In addition, as Dr. Kokelenberg was discussing and analyzing the cases, Roger van Zandvoort projected the MacRepertory/Complete Repertory analysis on a screen and demonstrated the use of the computer in case analysis. Mr. van Zandvoort's remarks, included wherever possible, are marked with his name and are also bracketed but not italicized.]

Case Number 1:
Anxious, Fastidious, and Obese

Female
Age 62

Initial Visit: August 17, 1993

Chief Complaints:
- Rheumatoid arthritis of both knees.
- Periarthritis scapulohumeralis (PSH) of her right shoulder (2).
- Rheumatic pains in her fingers.
- Deformed fingers.
- Cervicarthrosis.
- Spondylarthrosis.
- Epicondylitis radialis (tennis elbow) in her right arm (2).

[*Her most limiting complaints were the PSH and the tennis elbow.*]

Worse from exertion of joints.

Worse from cold air and cold, wet weather.

Joints crack on motion.

Stiffness when beginning to move.

Sometimes a cold sensation inside the joints.

Cannot stay immobile; has to keep on moving; restless.

[*In my experience, Rhus toxicodendron is deceiving in this kind of case. You frequently see these modalities, and Rhus toxicodendron almost never does anything of benefit. So, there must be other modalities for this remedy that are far more typical. Plus, some other remedies are more sensitive to cold and wet weather than Rhus toxicodendron. Dulcamara is one such remedy. We will see another in a moment.*]

Observations:

- Obese; hypertrophic mammae; protruding abdomen.
- Conglobated acne on her face, especially on the chin.
- Arthritic nodosities of many finger joints.
- Swollen thyroid gland (nodular goiter [cold nodule] right lower part; euthyroid, according to recent blood examination).

Height: 5 feet; weight 180 pounds.

Para: G4 P3 A1.

Even though obese, very chilly (even in a warm room).

Aversion to drafts and wind; takes cold easily.

[*She is quite chilly. I sometimes make house calls. When I go to her place, I have to remove my vest because it is so warm. It is like a sauna, but she feels comfortable there. She is very sensitive to drafts. Her husband jokes that if he opens his vest, she feels a draft!*]

Easily exhausted by the least physical exercise; perspires profusely all over.

Menopause since age 48, with severe climacteric flushes at night.

Feels completely exhausted after these flushes.

Pessary because of genital prolapse (uterine and vaginal) since her first pregnancy.

Strong palpitations with the least excitement.

High blood pressure (170/100); takes calcium antagonist medication every day.

Drinks about two quarts a day, especially warm drinks.

Her wounds and acne heal slowly because she cannot resist scratching the scars until they bleed.

Very constipated; takes laxatives every day.

Bites her nails.

Total dental prosthesis from the age of 32.

Scoliosis

Loves eggs and cheese. [This makes us think of Calcarea carbonica.]

Likes hot milk, hot soup, and alcohol [because these make her warm].

Craves fat, although she knows it is not good for her.

Hates cold drinks, ice, and ice cream.

Always lamenting about her health; pities herself; afraid she might become an invalid.
   [Calcarea carbonica is added in bold type for self-pity.]

Every symptom disturbs her peace.

[*It disturbs my peace, too (audience laughter)! The least suffering is too much for her. She wants immediate relief from every symptom. The worst thing that can happen to me is to go to the office on Monday morning and find that the first telephone call is from her. That can really lower my spirits. It is always, "I am sick again and I want..." I don't mean to make fun of her. This is part of her sickness, you see, but that is the effect it has on me. She used to call me three or four times per week. This is getting better now.*

I keep a card for each of the remedies. I write peculiar things on these cards. For instance, I write the effect the remedy has on me, as a person—how the patient who needs that remedy makes me feel. I also note how I found the remedy—what made me think of that remedy for those patients. This system helps me.]

Pessimistic; predicts the worst that can happen and it is always on her mind that fate can strike at any moment.

Many fears, especially when there is a possible connection with death (cancer, heart attack, stroke).

Horrified by everything that has to do with death (funerals, corpses, hospitals, undertakers, cemeteries, horror movies, rats and vermin, crucifixes).

[*Her main fears have to do with death. Patients do not always tell you that directly. For instance, she will tell me, "I have a fear of narrow places," and she means a coffin. "I have a fear of rats," and she means rats that eat your corpse. Everything that has to do with death absolutely horrifies her. She cannot view a body. She is afraid of it—the confrontation with death, hospitals, doctors, whatever.*

But, on the other hand, there is nothing she loves more than reading medical books. I learn a lot from visiting patients' homes. In her library, there are romances about doctors and nurses and so on. There are medical encyclopedias for lay people, things like that. She loves it, and she is afraid of it. These are not contradictory and alternating states. It is normal for people who have a fear of disease to love to read about it. That is why we all went to medical school (audience laughter).]

Cannot leave things out of place; her house is as clean as a clinic.

[*She is a very neat woman, very proper. She is clean, and her house is clean. Every book on the shelf has its particular spot. She is very meticulous about it. That was the thing that disturbed me a bit, because I couldn't match it to a remedy.*]

Afraid of infection.

Sedentary; watches television while sewing and knitting.

Her hands must be busy, but her body loves to rest.

Full of cares about her own household affairs, not so preoccupied with the world outside.

[*I know her parents. I have visited them, too, and they have told me a lot about her. She was a cheerful person once. She used to be the life of the house—laughing all the time, telling jokes. After the birth of her daughter (years ago), she became sad. Her daughter has a strange syndrome of paresis in her lower limbs. It has never been cured, and I think it must have been the source of the patient's sadness. She is a real "cocooner." That is also a Calcarea sign.*]

Assessment: The following rubrics were used:

- MIND, Pities, herself.
- MIND, Anxiety, health, about. [*This is underlined three times.*]
- MIND, Horrible things affect profoundly.
- EXTERNAL THROAT, Goiter.
- EXTREMITIES, Arthritic nodosities, finger joints.
- EXTREMITIES, Pain, shoulder, right.

- BACK, Curvature of spine.
- GENERALITIES, Obesity.
- FEMALE GENITALIA, Prolapsus, uterus.
- GENERALITIES, Food, desire, milk, hot.

Plan: Calcarea carbonica 200K, single dose.

[Roger van Zandvoort: I will explain an analysis method that you may not be aware of, even if you are familiar with the MacRepertory program. It is a method that may help you with some of your cases, although I don't know whether it will be of use in this particular case.

After putting in the symptoms, using only the Totality Analysis option, you can see that Calcarea carbonica is clearly the strongest remedy suggestion (Figure 1). I will assign the symptom of anxiety about health a value of "3" because you emphasized that.

To generate other remedy ideas you can click on the graph that shows you the six specific analysis structures that we have within the program (Figure 2). Then, look for the specific analyses that have the best "curves." By this, I mean the ones that have the best differentiation between the first and fifth remedies. Here you can see that we would select Strange, Rare, and Peculiar; Symptom Strength; and Keynotes.

Then go to the analysis menu and click on those strategies, at the same time removing the Totality Analysis option. Now you have a combination analysis with a different emphasis (Figure 3). As you can see, Calcarea carbonica still comes up highest, but other remedies are suggested for your consideration. This can be especially helpful if you give Calcarea carbonica and it doesn't work. You can return to this analysis and perhaps generate a new idea.]

Follow-Up on Case Number 1

September 21, 1993

Her constipation seems to be better.

Her climacteric disorders have improved.

Her rheumatic complaints are the same.

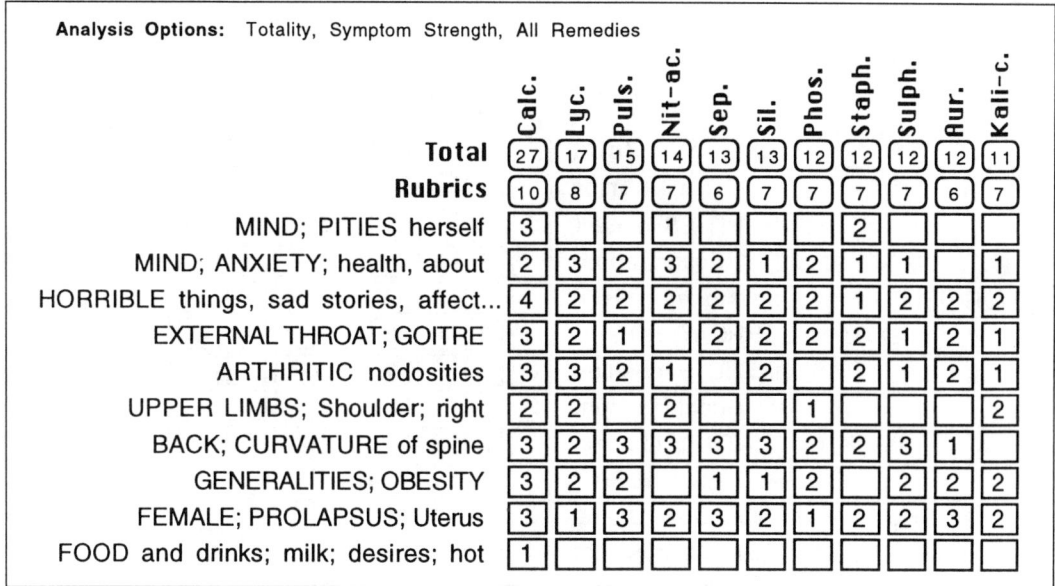

Analysis Options: Totality, Symptom Strength, All Remedies

	Calc.	Lyc.	Puls.	Nit-ac.	Sep.	Sil.	Phos.	Staph.	Sulph.	Aur.	Kali-c.
Total	27	17	15	14	13	13	12	12	12	12	11
Rubrics	10	8	7	7	6	7	7	7	7	6	7
MIND; PITIES herself	3			1				2			
MIND; ANXIETY; health, about	2	3	2	3	2	1	2	1	1		1
HORRIBLE things, sad stories, affect...	4	2	2	2	2	2	2	1	2	2	2
EXTERNAL THROAT; GOITRE	3	2	1		2	2	2	2	1	2	1
ARTHRITIC nodosities	3	3	2	1		2		2	1	2	1
UPPER LIMBS; Shoulder; right	2	2		2			1				2
BACK; CURVATURE of spine	3	2	3	3	3	3	2	2	3	1	
GENERALITIES; OBESITY	3	2	2		1	1	2		2	2	2
FEMALE; PROLAPSUS; Uterus	3	1	3	2	3	2	1	2	2	3	2
FOOD and drinks; milk; desires; hot	1										

Figure 1
Initial Totality Analysis for Case Number 1

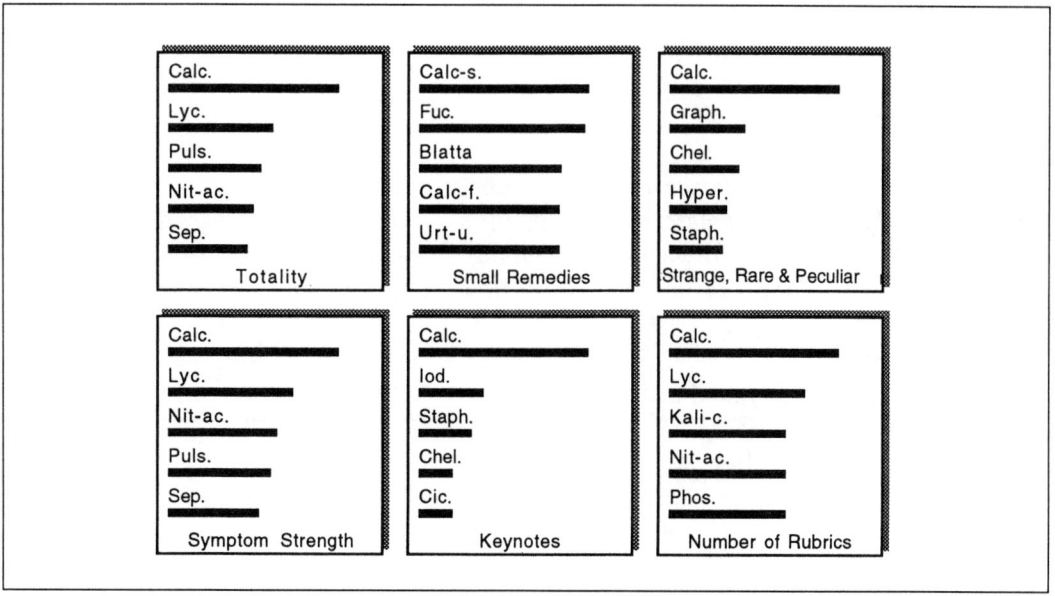

Figure 2
Initial Analysis Strategies for Case Number 1

Analysis Options: <u>Strange, Rare & Peculiar</u>, Symptom Strength, <u>Keynotes</u>, All Remedies

	Calc.	Staph.	Lyc.	Iod.	Nit-ac.	Puls.	Sep.	Graph.	Chel.	Phos.	Sil.
Total	27	12	17	10	14	15	13	11	5	12	13
Rubrics	10	7	8	6	7	7	6	5	3	7	7
MIND; PITIES herself	3	2			1						
MIND; ANXIETY; health, about	2	1	3		3	2	2			2	1
HORRIBLE things, sad stories, affect...	4	1	2	3	2	2	2			2	2
EXTERNAL THROAT; GOITRE	3	2	2	3		1	2	2		2	2
ARTHRITIC nodosities	3	2	3	1	1	2		3			2
UPPER LIMBS; Shoulder; right	2		2		2				3	1	
BACK; CURVATURE of spine	3	2	2	1	3	3	3			2	3
GENERALITIES; OBESITY	3		2	1		2	1	3		2	1
FEMALE; PROLAPSUS; Uterus	3	2	1	1	2	3	3	2	1	1	2
FOOD and drinks; milk; desires; hot	1							1	1		

Figure 3
First Combination Analysis for Case Number 1

Her blood pressure is worse (180/100).

Score: 3/10 to 5/10.

[*In the initial interview, I always ask my patients to give themselves a score that rates their general mental and physical state, with ten points as the highest possible score. After giving the remedy, I ask them to score themselves again. If they say "10," I write in my notes "liar" (audience laughter). In this instance, she went from "3" to "5," which is certainly possible.*]

Plan: 1. Wait.
2. Moderate physical exercise.
3. Physiotherapy.
4. Hypocaloric diet.

October 19, 1993

No improvement.

No new symptoms.

Her constipation has returned.

No more climacteric flushes.

Her PSH in her right shoulder and right tennis elbow are worse.

Score is back to 4/10.

Plan: Calcarea carbonica 200K, single dose.

October 27, 1993

No improvement.

According to an orthopedic specialist her PSH is worse and is moving toward a frozen shoulder situation.

Score is 3-4/10.

Assessment: The following rubrics were used:

- MIND, Rest, cannot, when things are not in proper place.
- MIND, Fastidious.
- MIND, Despair, recovery.
- MIND, Fear, cancer.
- MIND, Lamenting.
- CHEST, Palpitations, excitement of emotions, from.
- EXTERNAL THROAT, Goiter.
- GENERALITIES, Obesity.
- GENERALITIES, Cold, in general, aggravates.
- FEMALE GENITALIA, Menopause.
- FEMALE GENITALIA, Prolapsus, uterus.
- FEMALE GENITALIA, Prolapsus, vagina.
- GENERALITIES, Food, hot soup, desire for.
- GENERALITIES, Food, fats, desire for.
- GENERALITIES, Food, milk, warm, desire for.

Plan: Calcarea arsenica 200K, single dose.

[*She was not better. I felt nervous, which is the best thing that can happen to me. I re-evaluated the case and reviewed a few other rubrics. I was struck this time by how restless she was until everything was in order. I thought of the rubric, MIND, Rest, cannot, when things are not in proper place. This rubric indicates Arsenicum album and a few others (Anacardium, Arsenicum album, Aurum metallicum, Carcinosin, Sepia, Sulphur).*

If everything is not in its proper place, Arsenicum patients are afraid they will need something and won't be able to find it. It is the danger of not finding the thing in time. That is why everything has to be in order.

Carcinosin has the need to fulfill the things other people want from them. Their father or mother says, "You must put everything in order," and they feel bad if they don't do it.

Sepia's presence in this rubric has to do with its amelioration from occupation. Sepia must be occupied.

Sulphur is strange. What represents order for a Sulphur patient is not exactly order for the rest of us. Order is sort of an idea for Sulphur.

Because I thought this rubric was a bit too small, I also looked at the rubric, MIND, Fastidious.

The rubric for vaginal prolapse was interesting to me, because it is not as large as the one for uterine prolapse.

As I looked at the rubrics I had chosen (with repertory additions), I began to think of Calcarea arsenica. There were strong elements for Calcarea and strong elements for Arsenicum. The computer analysis, with the Totality Analysis option, demonstrates this (Figure 4). Calcarea arsenica has the desire for hot soup and covers the fastidious element better than Calcarea carbonica.

Boericke describes Calcarea arsenica as a remedy for fat women during menopause, with the "slightest emotion causing palpitation." So, I felt comfortable and prescribed the remedy.]

Analysis Options: Totality, All Remedies	Calc.	Sep.	Ars.	Puls.	Sulph.	Nux-v.	Phos.	Aur.	Nat-m.	Plat.	Graph.
Total	24	23	22	19	19	18	18	17	17	17	15
Rubrics	11	12	10	9	11	9	11	9	12	11	6
REST; cannot, when things are not in...		1	2		1		1		1		
MIND; FASTIDIOUS		1	2	3	1	2	1	1	2	1	2
MIND; DESPAIR; recovery	3	2	3	1	1	1	1		1	1	
MIND; FEAR; cancer, of	3	1	3				1		1	3	
LAMENTING, bemoaning, wailing	2	1	2	2	2	2	1	3	1	1	
PALPITATION heart; excitement, after	1	2	2	2		2	3	2	1	2	
EXTERNAL THROAT; GOITRE	3	2		1	1		2	2	2	1	2
GENERALITIES; OBESITY	3	1	2	2	2		2	2	2	1	3
GENERALITIES; COLD; agg.	3	3	3	2	2	3	3	2	2	1	3
FEMALE; MENOPAUSE	1	3		3	3	2	2	1	1	2	3
FEMALE; PROLAPSUS; Uterus	3	3	2	3	2	2	1	3	2	3	2
FEMALE; PROLAPSUS; Vagina		3				2	2			1	
FOOD and drinks; soup; desires; warm									1		
FOOD and drinks; fats and rich food;...	1		1		2	2	1		1		
FOOD and drinks; milk; desires; warm	1										

Figure 4
Second Totality Analysis for Case Number 1

[Roger van Zandvoort: If we pursue the approach that I described earlier using this new combination of rubrics, we can see that the Small Remedies and perhaps the Strange, Rare, and Peculiar strategies now show the kind of curve we would select (Figure 5). Whenever you change one or more rubrics, it creates an entirely new constellation that requires a fresh analysis. Now we see that Calcarea arsenica comes up strongly (Figure 6).]

[*When the small remedies are emphasized, we see Carcinosin coming to the forefront. This is probably her nosode, but she doesn't need it at this time.*]

Totality	Small Remedies	Strange, Rare & Peculiar
Calc.	Calc-ar.	Calc.
Sep.	Carc.	Bry.
Ars.	Aur-s.	Chel.
Puls.	Thyr.	Nat-m.
Sulph.	Lob.	Ars.

Symptom Strength	Keynotes	Number of Rubrics
Calc.	Ars.	Nat-m.
Sep.	Calc.	Sep.
Ars.	Sep.	Calc.
Puls.	Puls.	Phos.
Sulph.	Calc-ar.	Plat.

Figure 5
Second Analysis Strategies for Case Number 1

Analysis Options: <u>Small Remedies, Strange, Rare & Peculiar</u>, All Remedies

	Calc-ar.	Carc.	Aur-s.	Plat.	Thyr.	Kali-ar.	Lob.	Ferr.	Lycps.	Aur.	Fuc.
Total	15	11	9	17	8	10	7	14	6	17	4
Rubrics	9	8	6	11	4	6	5	8	4	9	2
REST; cannot, when things are not in...		1								1	
MIND; FASTIDIOUS		3		1		2	2			1	
MIND; DESPAIR; recovery	1	1	2	1	2	1					
MIND; FEAR; cancer, of		1		3		2	2				
LAMENTING, bemoaning, wailing	1		1	1		1				3	
PALPITATION heart; excitement, after	2		1	2				1	2	2	
EXTERNAL THROAT; GOITRE		1	1	1	2			1	2	2	2
GENERALITIES; OBESITY	2	1		1	2		1	3	1	2	2
GENERALITIES; COLD; agg.	3		1	1	2	3	1	3	1	2	
FEMALE; MENOPAUSE	2	1		2				1		1	
FEMALE; PROLAPSUS; Uterus	1		3	3		1		2		3	
FEMALE; PROLAPSUS; Vagina	1			1				2			
FOOD and drinks; soup; desires; warm	2							1			
FOOD and drinks; fats and rich food;...		2					1				
FOOD and drinks; milk; desires; warm											

Figure 6
Second Combination Analysis for Case Number 1

December 7, 1993

The rheumatic pains in her right shoulder and right elbow are much better.

Her stools are much easier.

No climacteric flushes.

Her blood pressure dropped to 140/90 at half the dose of her Ca-antagonistic drug.

Her acne is better.

She feels hopeful now and engages herself in social work.

Score is now 7-8/10.

Plan: Wait.

January 26, 1994

She noticed a yellow leucorrhoea.

Her Pap smear was Class III. This frightened her, because of her strong fear of cancer.

Within a week she relapsed: constipated, pain in right shoulder, lamenting about her bad luck.

Plan: Calcarea arsenica 200K, single dose.

February 8, 1994

After the remedy she had a flu for about a week and was prescribed placebo granules.

She feels fine again.

Plan: Wait.

April 7, 1994

A control review of the Pap smear was Class II.

She continues to feel fine.

She stopped taking her blood pressure medication; her blood pressure remained 140/90.

No more constipation when she eats rye bread and fruit.

She can do mild physical exercise without feeling exhausted now.

Her weight is now 167 pounds after a diet.

Her relatives say she is more lively and less pessimistic.

Her PSH has improved; mobility is better; pain is much less.

No more discomfort in her right elbow.

Plan: Wait.

This patient has remained very well to the present.

Case Number 2:
"I Never Succeed in Anything"

Female
Age 29

This case was an intriguing one. First of all, the pathology is difficult. Anorexia nervosa is a very difficult pathology. Second, I felt compassion for her, which made it more difficult for me.

Initial Visit: October 10, 1992

Chief Complaints:
- Anorexia nervosa.
- Secondary amenorrhea.

- Severe constipation; uses laxatives.
- Dry, itching eczema in axillae.
- Recurrent herpetic eruptions under the nose.
- Muscae volitantes.

She was the first of seven children.

Her mother became pregnant with the patient and married because of the pregnancy.

At age 22 the patient married a man she loves.

The anorexia began when she was a child, but it is out of control now.

Feels forsaken by her mother. She thinks her mother hates her because she was forced into marriage.

Projects the same forsaken feeling in her relations with her husband, her mother-in-law, and her sister.

[*I met her mother, who does have some resentment about having to marry. Her marriage is not happy. But the mother's resentment is not that severe. My patient says, "My mother doesn't like me. She neglects me and deserts me." But that isn't really true. It is an illusion. She really believes her mother hates her. She does the same thing toward her husband, who loves and adores her.*]

Introverted, reserved, and timid. She wants to hide her feelings because she doesn't want to be hurt. Silent grief.

Wanted to be a perfect child.

Very severe with herself. Avoids the possibility of being criticized. No self-confidence.

Feels better at home. Avoids company. Aversion to going out.

[*"Aversion to going out" reminds me of another small remedy that has this symptom. I treated a boy who had a dust allergy. He looked like a Chamomilla. But he had this same symptom, which is exactly the opposite of Chamomilla. Chamomilla wants to go out, is restless, wants to leave the house, and so on. I was a bit puzzled. He had a cough resulting from the allergy. Every time he entered the house, he had a cough. When he was out, it was better.*

So I had these two symptoms, aversion to going out and coughing on entering a warm room. I gave him Anthemis nobilis, which is "Roman chamomile." Look for it in Boericke. It is a Chamomilla who doesn't want to go out. This has nothing to do with this case (audience laughter).]

Afraid of cancer and impending serious diseases. Afraid of dying.

Observation: She talks very loudly and with excitement. Loquacious. She gives the impression that she is tense. She is not relaxed during the interview.

Brittle nails.

Thin hair, falling diffusely.

Wounds heal slowly.

Very chilly, but cannot stand the sun.

Habitual constipation, but gets diarrhea after drinking coffee.

Herpes under her nose.

Assessment: The following rubrics were used:

- MIND, Ailments, grief, after.
- MIND, Grief, silent.
- MIND, Homesickness.
- FACE, Eruptions, herpes, nose.
- GENERALITIES, Sun, exposure to, aggravates.
- RECTUM, Diarrhea, coffee, after.

Plan: Natrum muriaticum 1,000K, single dose.

Follow-Up on Case Number 2

November 30, 1992

She felt very tired immediately after taking the remedy; sleepy all day.

She had a migraine-type headache the second day after the remedy. The pain was relieved somewhat when she tried to draw her eyes together as in convergent strabismus (Kent, page 238).

She feels terribly angry inside, directed particularly toward her mother. She demands a remedy for the anger to avoid quarrels.

Her axillary eczema is worse.

Plan: 1. Placebo.
      2. Calendula talc, externally.
      3. Wait.

March 31, 1993

She had a problem with her mother-in-law. (This may be her first step toward confronting her own mother.) She feels humiliated by her, hates her, feels ugly, and feels laughed at.

Her axillary eczema is better, but it itches severely now.

She avoids the sight of people. She weeps when nobody can see her.

Plan: Natrum muriaticum 1,000K, single dose.

April 21, 1993

After taking the remedy her mood was changeable. Some days were good; some were miserable.

Her menses started again yesterday (last menses eight months ago).

Her hair is better now.

Her constipation is so bad that her anus prolapses during a stool.

She feels very sad now, to the point of committing suicide.

"The only thing I am really good at is refusing myself the pleasure of eating and drinking."

"My mother is the most important theme in my life."

"I am afraid of undertaking anything. I never succeed in anything. I am a coward. I lack the courage to get started."

She is very discontented with herself.

"When I am occupied I feel better."

Assessment: The anger toward her mother indicates a muriatic remedy. Natrum muriaticum gave slight improvement, produced changeable moods, and brought back her menses. But she still suppresses her feelings toward her mother. The picture of an anorexic person for me is a combination of physical weakness, because of starvation, and tremendous willpower to accomplish the weight loss at the same time. The weakness suggests an acid. I read in a Dutch magazine about the fear of failure associated with a lesser-known muriatic remedy.

At this point, I used the following rubrics (Figure 7):

- MIND, Sadness, menses, during.
- MIND, Cowardice.
- MIND, Confidence, want of self.
- MIND, Occupation, ameliorates.
- RECTUM, Prolapsus, stool, during.

Plan: Muriaticum acidum 200K, single dose.

May 26, 1993

The change in her stools was the first sign of improvement. She now has a stool every other day without the help of any laxatives.

Her menses came on May 23 and is very painful.

The axillary eczema is still there, but the itching is less.

	Calc.	Ign.	Lyc.	Mur-ac.	Aur.	Lach.	Merc.	Nat-c.	Nat-m.	Nit-ac.	Nux-v.	Puls.
Total	6	8	10	5	5	5	4	5	6	4	7	7
Rubrics	5	5	5	5	4	4	4	4	4	4	4	4
SADNESS, despondency, dejection,...	1	1	1	1	1		1	1	2	1		2
MIND; COWARDICE	1	1	3	1	1	1	1		1	1	2	2
MIND; CONFIDENCE; want of self	1	1	2	1	2	1	1	1	2	1	1	2
OCCUPATION, diversion; amel.	1	2	1	1	1	1		2			2	1
RECTUM; PROLAPSE; stool; during	2	3	3	1		2	1	1	1	1	2	

Analysis Options: Number of Rubrics, All Remedies

Figure 7
Final Repertorization for Case Number 2

She feels that her self-confidence has dramatically improved. She made the appointment on her own to see me this time. She also took driving lessons, and she went to the dentist.

She said she feels better than she did after taking the Natrum muriaticum because her condition is more stable.

The only time she felt sad was before her menses.

Plan: Wait.

[*This is new information. Muriatic acid has the delusion that they cannot succeed, the fear of failure: "I am not good for anything. I can't do anything. I cannot succeed. I will fail." Muriatic acid is not under the rubric, MIND, Delusion, cannot succeed, does everything wrong. Nor is it under MIND, Fear, failure, of. It is listed under MIND, Confidence, want of self, and under MIND, Succeeds, never.*]

June 6, 1993

She finally had the courage to talk with her mother yesterday about her feelings toward her. They had a terrible argument.

She didn't sleep well last night.

Herpes appeared under her nose today.

She says she will have a nervous breakdown.

Plan: Placebo, because she actually looked quite satisfied to me.

September 21, 1993

She is in excellent condition.

No more constipation. She has a stool every two days.

Her menses are regular and painless; flow is normal.

Her eczema has disappeared.

Her appetite is good, but she still has a distended feeling after meals.

Plan: Wait.

Long-Term Follow-Up

She has continued to do very well, with only the one initial dose of Muriatic acid 200K.

She has gained weight.

Her stools are normal.

She is working.

She is going out.

She is driving.

She has made peace with her mother. She spoke out her feelings, and everything was all right.

[*I was very pleased with the result in this case. Since then, I have had three more cases of anorexia nervosa that I treated successfully with Muriatic acid.*]

[Roger van Zandvoort: This was a case that really could not be solved using Kent's repertory or the Complete Repertory, so we still have some work to do.]

The Complete Repertory: How it Came into Being
(Roger van Zandvoort)

Originally, I simply wanted to have a better repertory for myself. Many other people have probably done something similar over the years. I have always been a collector. In the past, I collected butterflies. Now I take photographs of them! Later on, I collected cacti.

About ten years ago, I became more professionally interested in this work. I was busily entering Vithoulkas' additions, those compiled by Bill Gray, into the *Synthetic Repertory*. What I saw was that there were many additions that were not in the *Synthetic Repertory*. I felt these really should be added. Also, some of Vithoulkas' additions in the *Synthetic Repertory* were in different degrees. So, which one was right?

The only way to find out is to consult the homeopathic materia medica. In doing that, I found many more remedies that could and should be added into those rubrics. So, the *Synthetic Repertory* was not a complete repertory. This was a disappointment for me.

It was then that I began to investigate systematically what the additions to the repertory should be, as well as what corrections needed to be made. If you search the old homeopathic journals carefully, especially the *Homeopathic Recorder*, you will find a number of corrections for Kent's repertory compiled by Kent's students. For example, in 1924 there were many corrections published by Pugh. Not too many people know about that. It is nice to see that kind of work, although we should always check the corrections against the materia medica.

Kent used part of Allen's index—the last two volumes of the 12 volumes of Allen's encyclopedia—to build his repertory. Allen added the index because the ten volumes of materia medica, a massive amount of information, needed cross-referencing. There are quite a few mistakes in this index. I think Allen had difficulty reading his own handwriting in later years. Kent then carried Allen's errors over to the repertory.

You can imagine how things might have gone wrong. Think about the similarity of abbreviations for Chlorum (Chlor.), Chloralum (Chlol.), and Chloroform (Chlf.). It was not hard to mix them up. In Allen's index, for example, you will find the abbreviation for Chlorum under the symptom of shrieking. It should have been Chloralum.

Under dreams of insects, you will find Spigelia (Spig.). This should have been Sphingurus (Sphing.), which is a kind of Brazilian porcupine. There are more of these instances for Spigelia.

You will find Opium under the main rubric for cursing, and also under cursing in the afternoon and in the evening, when at home. The remedy should have been Opuntia vulgaris, the prickly pear. If you check in Allen's materia medica, you will see that these are symptoms for Opuntia vulgaris. Nearly all the repertories took up these mistakes. Later on, Opium was added in its own right by Gallavardin into the main rubric for cursing.

There are many such errors, too many to mention. We are correcting them as we find them. I currently have 40 people working on additions and corrections for the Complete Repertory.

My life became a lot easier when David Warkentin (of Kent Homeopathic Associates) created ReferenceWorks, which is a wonderful tool. I use it constantly to search for precise, in-depth information about what to add to the Complete Repertory. This is how you can find the discrepancies between Allen's materia medica and his index. Both works are in ReferenceWorks and, by comparing the two, you can discover the discrepancies.

I have also frequently used Guy Kokelenberg's (and Dr. Dockx's) *Comparative Materia Medica* in my work. It is very helpful. I think Guy's greatest strength is his ability to differentiate clearly between specific remedies in a given rubric, and this is part of what his book provides. It also has many cross-references for rubrics, and we have used these in the Complete Repertory.

Case Number 3:
Convinced She Is Ugly

Female
Age 34

Initial Visit: December 4, 1991

Chief Complaint: Generalized psoriasis; dry, glistening red, itching, 3-to-5-cm patches. It began before puberty, was treated with Mopsoralene, ultraviolet light, and cortisone ointments. It disappeared almost completely until after her first pregnancy.

Family History:

- Father: Psoriasis; died suddenly of an acute myocardial infarction.
- Mother: Pulmonary tuberculosis as a child; developed asthma afterwards; died during patient's second pregnancy of a Grawitz tumor (renal cancer).
- Sister (older): Drinking problem.
- Brothers (two, younger): Healthy.

Two consecutive spontaneous abortions, each one after bad news (her dog died; her mother was diagnosed with cancer).

[*I must make a comment about something Anne Schadde said yesterday. She said that the reaction a person has toward a given stressor is the most important element in finding the remedy because it reflects the individual. I agree. On the other hand, I disagree, too, because I think that etiologies and our susceptibilities to them have something to do with our individuality. We are confronted in life with those things that have something to teach us. For this reason, I always like to see the remedy I prescribe in the appropriate etiological rubric, because that etiology must have something to do with that remedy. In this case, for example, she must have some susceptibility to bad news, because she had spontaneous abortions after hearing of these things.*]

The psoriasis was worse after each pregnancy.

Para: G4 P2 A2.

Suffered a truncal herpes zoster eruption during her first lactation period. Breast-feeding therefore had to be stopped.

Recurrent herpes simplex around her mouth.

Headaches from exposure to the sun and after fasting.

Sleeps on her abdomen. She perspires as she's falling asleep.

During winter her hands are deeply cracked.

Has a tendency to get colds, suppurative conjunctivitis, and sinusitis frontalis as a common complication of coryza.

Neck pain and torticollis after exposure to cold, wet weather and drafts.

Dislikes sweets, but craves them on rare occasions.

Desires fatty, salty, spicy foods.

The psoriasis is like a stigma for her. She hates it, she thinks it makes her ugly, and she believes her husband thinks that she is ugly and would never have married her if he had known that she had psoriasis.

[*Actually, she is quite beautiful. Her husband adores her and accepts her psoriasis without a second thought.*]

She is a bookkeeper and is well respected for her work.

[*I know her boss, who is also my patient. He told me she is quite good and is greatly appreciated. Yet, she always has the feeling that everyone is looking down on her.*]

Closed, reserved, taciturn.

After a quarrel she will be mocking and will brood for days without speaking a word.

[*She can be quite angry. I experienced her anger once.*]

When sad, she retires and weeps alone. Does not want to be helped or consoled by anyone.

Afraid of the dark as a child. Looked under the bed for robbers. Even now, she doesn't feel comfortable alone in the dark. Always takes the dog with her.

Everything must be done in a hurry; everybody must hurry.

Assessment: The following rubrics were used:

- MIND, Grief, ailments from.
- MIND, Mortification, ailments from.
- MIND, Bad news, ailments from.
- MIND, Hurry.
- MIND, Reserved.
- MIND, Consolation aggravates.
- FACE, Eruptions, herpes, lips, about.
- GENERALITIES, Food, salt, desire for.

Plan: Natrum muriaticum 200K, single dose.

Follow-Up on Case Number 3

April 2, 1991

Acute consultation.

For the past four months she has felt much better.

The psoriasis patches regressed. No more itching.

No more herpes.

Now she has a fever of 101°F; feels hot all over. Also she wants fresh air, she has a herpes simplex on the lower lip, her mouth feels dry but she doesn't drink more, and she has a sore throat when she swallows.

Recently she saw a program on television concerning skin diseases and psoriasis. Since then, she has been feeling depressed again, cannot sleep, quit her job without any reason, and doesn't want to leave her house.

She is afraid her children will get psoriasis. One of them has slight eczema but no psoriasis.

Her psoriasis patches start to itch and burn, and she says new ones develop every day.

Assessment: The psoriasis subsided, but the constitution was not in order. The last four months she felt much better, no more itching, but then she came in for an acute consultation. These were Apis symptoms. Apis is the acute of Natrum muriaticum, so I felt good about prescribing it. I told her afterwards to repeat Natrum muriaticum. This acute episode came after she saw a television program concerning psoriasis, which was a kind of bad news.

The following rubrics were used:

- MIND, Bad news, ailments from.
- SKIN, Eruptions, burning.
- FEVER, Uncovering, desire for.
- STOMACH, Thirstless, heat, during.
- MOUTH, Dryness, thirstless.

Plan: Apis mellifica 200K, single dose.

September 25, 1991

She comes in with her husband.

Within one day after the remedy the fever disappeared.

Within a few days the herpes healed.

Her condition has returned to normal, but the psoriasis has remained the same and her emotional state is unstable.

Her husband asked for this consultation because they are having serious problems in their relationship.

She is very jealous and irritable. She says he sees other women. Feels abandoned by him. Envies him because her parents died and his parents are alive.

[*There is absolutely no basis for her jealousy. Her husband adores her and constantly reassures her.*]

(During the consultation she gets very upset and leaves without a word.)

He says that she consumes too much alcohol and he is afraid she will develop a drinking habit like her older sister.

(After a while she returns and I ask her husband to leave the room.)

She believes that everyone is looking at her and that she looks ugly. She stays indoors and closes the curtains.

[*The fear of being observed is a Calcarea element. The fear of being observed because she feels ugly is the state of Calcarea sulphurica.*]

The psoriasis is worse. It burns, and the patches are very red.

She perspires, and her axillary perspiration has an offensive odor.

Has a strong desire for sweets now.

[*This is a new symptom. It is interesting that during this acute situation, she has a strong desire for sweets. I believe food desires and aversions, if they are very strong, should be elevated in the hierarchy, right under the mental symptoms. This is because they have to do with the mental state. You see, life isn't sweet enough, so she crave sweets.*]

Assessment: Apis was suppressive. Now I was able to see her state clearly. The following rubrics were used (Figure 8):

- MIND, Forsaken feeling.
- MIND, Quarrelsomeness.
- MIND, Jealousy.
- MIND, Lamenting, appreciated, because she is not.
- SKIN, Eruptions, psoriasis.
- SKIN, Eruptions, burning.
- GENERALITIES, Food, sweets, desires.

Plan: Calcarea sulphurica 200K, single dose.

Analysis Options: Number of Rubrics, All Remedies	Calc-s.	Calc.	Kali-c.	Nat-m.	Plat.	Puls.	Sep.	Alum.	Anac.
Total	9	7	8	7	9	10	8	4	5
Rubrics	6	5	5	5	5	5	5	4	4
MIND; FORSAKEN feeling	1	1	1	2	2	3	1	1	1
MIND; QUARRELSOMENESS, scolding	1	1	2	2	2	1	2	1	2
MIND; JEALOUSY	2	1	1	1	3	2	1		1
LAMENTING, bemoaning, wailing; appreciated,...	1								
SKIN; ERUPTIONS; psoriasis	2	2	2	1	1	2	3	1	
SKIN; ERUPTIONS; painful; burning	2	2	2	1	1	2	1	1	1

Figure 8
Final Repertorization for Case Number 3

March 25, 1992

She and her husband saw a therapist for their relationship. She feels happy in her marriage again.

She went back to work and feels satisfied with her job.

No more psoriasis, except for two patches on her elbows.

She complains of coryza with a sore throat and slight fever.

Assessment: Calcarea sulphurica is the correct remedy.

Plan: 1. Placebo.
       2. Phytogargarism (herbal gargle).
       3. Vitamin C.

May 29, 1992

Acute consultation.

She and her husband had an argument, and her psoriasis is coming back in small spots on her trunk.

Plan: Calcarea sulphurica 200K, single dose.

April 28, 1993

She has had no problems for about a year.

Complains of a cervicalgia after exposure to a cold wind. Local physiotherapy and painkillers did not help. She took a dose of the last remedy on her own a week ago, and it did not help either.

Plan: Calcarea phosphorica 200K, single dose.

November 3, 1993

She feels depressed.

Suffers from continuous nausea and headaches.

Her psoriasis has reappeared.

She went to the cemetery to visit her parents' graves.

Assessment: Calcarea phosphorica, although well indicated, was suppressive.

Plan: Calcarea sulphurica 200K, single dose.

February 11, 1994

Complains of coryza with a sore throat.

No more problems.

She feels happy.

The psoriasis is on her elbows only.

Plan: 1. Placebo.
2. Phytogargarism.
3. Vitamin C.

Case Number 4:
His Mother Does the Talking

Male
Age 19

Initial Visit: March 17, 1993

Chief Complaints: Allergic skin disease. His skin itches, without any apparent eruption. Mostly occurs in the axillary, groin, head, and perineum regions. It is worse in warm weather and when he becomes heated.

[*The itching is worse from everything that provokes heat—alcohol, exercise, warm baths, eating warm food, the sun. If you really think about this initial information you already have the remedy. But we don't usually think that clearly. After I had found the remedy, I realized that he had told me the remedy from the beginning!*]

On further interrogation, I discover that he is on Asacol (mesalazine), four tablets a day. He is taking it for ileitis terminalis (Crohn's disease), which was diagnosed during puberty when he was suffering from diarrhea and severe anemia.

[*He came to see me for the allergic dermatitis. During the interview I asked him if he had any other problems. He said he didn't, but when I asked him if he took any medicine he mentioned the Asacol for Crohn's disease! He thought of this as "normal." The doctor had told him he had Crohn's disease and that he should learn to live with it. So, he took his Asacol regularly and from time to time needed steroid enemas. For him, it was normal.*]

This young man always comes accompanied by his mother. He is not that young, 19 years old, yet she does much of the talking. It seems to irritate him, but he doesn't do anything about it. He just grimaces from time to time when she isn't looking.

[*He is slender, red-haired, with many freckles. When he shakes your hand, his hand is limp— a "blubber hand." I always shake my patient's hand, as a first piece of information. Some patients have hot hands, some have cold hands, and some have sweaty hands that are either cold or warm. Some Lycopodium patients have you on your knees with the firmness of their*] *handshake! Other patients with arthritic nodosities go on their knees when you shake their hand (audience laughter)! Anyway, he had cold, sweaty, clammy hands. He had myopia, and his glasses were so thick that he must have had good eyes to see through them (audience laughter)!]*

Frequent pseudocroup attacks at night as a little child.

Recurrent otitis media as a child. Transtympanal drains for impaired hearing.

Severe pains in the bones of his legs at night for some time; diagnosed as growing pains. Is not having the pains at the moment.

[All of these symptoms are indications for the remedy, including the growing pains, but I didn't see it at this point.]

Family History:
- Father: Otosclerosis.
- Paternal Aunt: Juvenile diabetes.
- Mother: Highly allergic.
- Maternal Grandfather: Died of leukemia.
- Maternal Grandmother: Died of lung cancer.

Rather chilly. Catches cold easily when the weather is cold and damp.

[The remedy for this case is the other remedy to remember for aggravation from cold and wet weather. There is Rhus toxicodendron, there is Dulcamara, and there is this remedy.]

Every coryza is complicated by bronchitis; takes antibiotics.

Perspires a lot in warm weather or in a warm room.

Red-haired, pale face, and pale lips.

[The presence of the pale lips means the anemia is still there, although he is taking Asacol, the intermittent steroids, and lots of iron supplements. Strangely enough, his remedy is closely related to iron.]

Allergic to dust; allergic rhinitis sets in after exposure.

Voice becomes husky when he talks too much.

Strong myopia of both eyes.

Loves chocolate.

Very thirsty for cold drinks, especially cold milk. Drinks two to three quarts a day.

Talks a lot; even talks in his sleep.

Many friends.

Shy.

His normally pale face turns red when he has to answer a question or when he takes a public shower.

Worries about accidents, diseases, fire, and war.

Plays classical guitar as a hobby.

[*It is not enough to ask people if they like music. You must also ask what kind of music. What do they listen to? Listen to it and try to catch the emotion that is coming out of this music. Then you will know something about the person. He loves classical guitar music. This is the kind of music that makes him cheerful.*]

Assessment: The following rubrics were used:

- MIND, Timidity, bashful.
- MIND, Talking, sleep, in.
- MIND, Anticipation, complaints, from.
- GENERALITIES, Anemia.
- STOMACH, Thirst, large quantities, for.
- FACE, Discoloration, pale.
- FACE, Discoloration, changing color.
- LARYNX, Voice, hoarseness, talking, from.
- GENERALITIES, Food, milk, cold, desire for.
- VISION, Myopia.

Plan: Phosphorus 200K, single dose.

Follow-Up on Case Number 4

April 7, 1993

Nothing happened after the remedy.

The itching is still the same.

Assessment: I concluded that the drug he was taking was antidotal and decided to give him LM potencies to be taken daily until a reaction occurred.

Plan: Phosphorus 0/2, one drop a day in a teaspoon of water after shaking the bottle.

April 20, 1993

Acute consultation.

During school examinations he caught a cold. He visited a physician, was diagnosed with bronchitis, and was prescribed antibiotics.

No amelioration came after three days, so he came to me for advice.

He was coughing severely. It was a barking cough, which was worse when he was outside in the rain. It disappeared at night.

His voice was hoarse.

He had sharp pain in the larynx.

No signs of bronchitis at this time.

His temperature is normal.

Assessment: There are no signs of bronchitis. It is probably a coryza complicated by laryngitis. I used the following rubrics (Figure 9):

- COUGH, Daytime, only.
- COUGH, Weather, damp.
- LARYNX, Inflammation.

- MIND, Fear, happen, something will.
- MIND, Timidity, bashful.
- GENERALITIES, Milk, desire for.
- VISION, Myopia.
- SKIN, Itching, perspiring parts.
- GENERALITIES, Feather bed aggravates.
- EXTREMITIES, Lower limbs, leg, growing pains.
- HEARING, Impaired, catarrh of eustachian tube.
- GENERALITIES, Anemia.

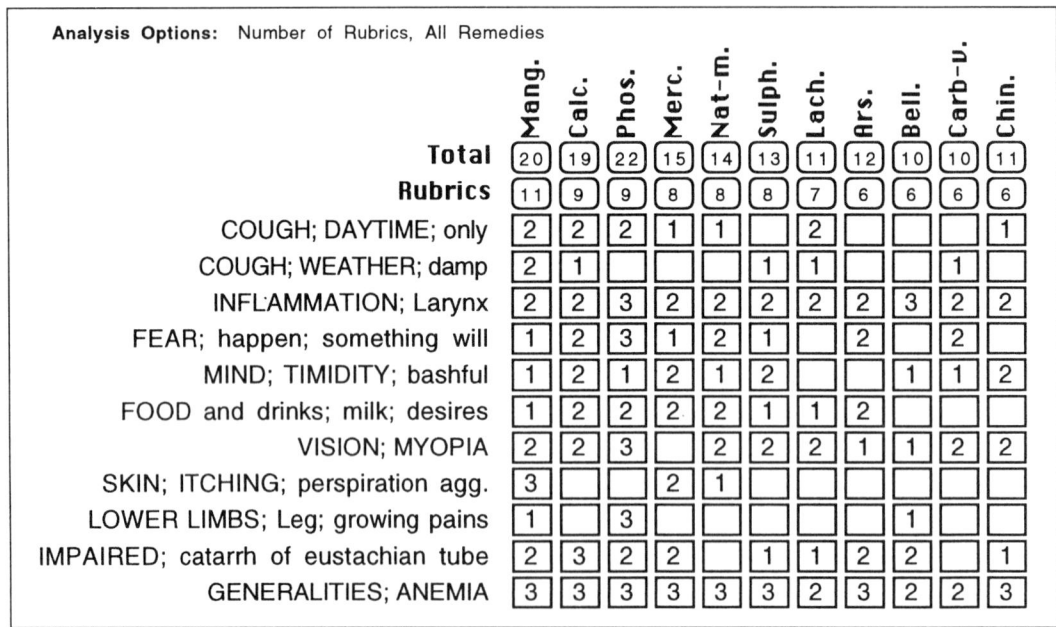

Analysis Options: Number of Rubrics, All Remedies

	Mang.	Calc.	Phos.	Merc.	Nat-m.	Sulph.	Lach.	Ars.	Bell.	Carb-v.	Chin.
Total	20	19	22	15	14	13	11	12	10	10	11
Rubrics	11	9	9	8	8	8	7	6	6	6	6
COUGH; DAYTIME; only	2	2	2	1	1		2				1
COUGH; WEATHER; damp	2	1				1	1			1	
INFLAMMATION; Larynx	2	2	3	2	2	2	2	2	3	2	2
FEAR; happen; something will	1	2	3	1	2	1		2		2	
MIND; TIMIDITY; bashful	1	2	1	2	1	2			1	1	2
FOOD and drinks; milk; desires	1	2	2	2	2	1	1	2			
VISION; MYOPIA	2	2	3		2	2	2	1	1	2	2
SKIN; ITCHING; perspiration agg.	3			2	1						
LOWER LIMBS; Leg; growing pains	1		3						1		
IMPAIRED; catarrh of eustachian tube	2	3	2	2		1	1	2	2		1
GENERALITIES; ANEMIA	3	3	3	3	3	3	2	3	2	2	3

Figure 9
Final Repertorization for Case Number 4

I used the rubric, MIND, Fear, happen, something will, instead of anticipation. And I used the aggravation from a feather bed because his dust allergy was mainly in bedrooms and he slept on a feather bed. (His mother is Austrian.) I also incorporated some old symptoms into the repertorization, such as growing pains and eustachian deafness.

I had serious doubts about the initial remedy. I thought that if I could treat the acute it would probably have a positive influence on his chronic condition as well, so I put more weight on the acute symptoms.

Plan: 1. Manganum 200K, single dose.
2. Phytotherapeutic syrup.
3. Stop antibiotics.

August 20, 1993

(He comes alone for the follow-up, for the first time.)

He rapidly felt better after the remedy.

His skin problem never came back.

Surprisingly, his Asacol therapy could be reduced and later stopped completely because his stools, sedimentation rate, and anemic parameters became normal.

Long-Term Follow-Up

He came to see me in April 1994 because he developed a hay fever attack from the nervous strain associated with his school examinations. I repeated the dose of Manganum 200K and everything was back to normal once again.

Manganum has produced a remarkable result in this case. I was very pleased. Crohn's disease, as you know, is a difficult disease to treat. He discontinued the Asacol on his own, because he felt so much better.

If you study Manganum, you will see that it covers his state well. It has the sensitivity to cold and wet, the anemia, the recurrent croup, the eustachian catarrh, and the growing pains. It has been added to the Complete Repertory, from Boericke, for the growing pains (EXTREMITY PAIN, Lower limbs, leg, growing pains).

It is close to Ferrum (iron), standing next to it in the periodic table of elements. It shares the anemia, the iron deficiency, with Ferrum. When I was studying this case, I also read what Rajan Sankaran has to say about Manganum in his book, *The Substance of Homeopathy.* I recommend that you look at it. Sankaran describes Manganum as very similar to Ferrum, in terms of being dominated and suppressed. The suppression is something like Carcinosin. The description mentions a shy child of dominating parents, a mild person with a yielding disposition. This description fits my patient very well.

Stephen King: Could you say a bit more about the phenomenon of finding the remedy from an acute circumstance? What is happening in an acute?

Kokelenberg: Things become more clear. The confusion is less. The symptoms are clearer. Mental symptoms are qualities of a person. But are they "symptoms"? I don't know. I think a mental symptom is a symptom that is disturbing the patient in his surroundings, and this becomes more clear in an acute. The general symptoms, too—desires and aversions—as well as the physical symptoms become more clear.

We get a spotlight on the patient's state. If you have the opportunity to treat acutes, the constitutional remedy often comes to the surface. Or, alternatively, the acute has something to do with the constitutional remedy. You find an Apis acute, and the constitutional remedy is Natrum muriaticum. You find a Belladonna acute, and the constitutional remedy is Calcarea carbonica. The acute case points you toward something significant. It has helped me frequently.

In addition, I think it has something to do with ourselves, the prescribers, because the acute gives you a kind of anxiety. I need that sort of excitement. Otherwise, I can become too lazy. Day after day, I am just sitting there with patients. With the acute—pneumonia or appendicitis—you are very excited. Coffea enters your body (audience laughter), and the mind becomes focused. I think it is a combination of all these factors.

Roger van Zandvoort: In the Chenopodium anthelminticum case, you were thinking about Lycopodium and Chelidonium originally. When you have such a case and then get a hint for a small remedy like Chenopodium, you can go to the Relationships of Remedies section of the Complete Repertory. There you can check to see if the small remedy has any connection with the other remedies you have previously been considering.

In the Relationships of Remedies section, click on the small remedy and then click on the Similar Action category. There you will find remedies that are known to be similar in action to the small remedy. Much of this information comes from Knerr's repertory, which has a big section on the relationship of remedies. Under Chenopodium anthelminticum, for example, the Similar Action category reveals that Lycopodium and Chelidonium are similar to Chenopodium (Figure 10). So, this is one useful way to check the connection between remedies.

Chenopodium
anthelminthicum, Worm-seed, North America, Central

RELATIONSHIPS

Families Chenopodium: chen-a., chen-v.
Similar action: aphis.$_2$, chel.$_2$, chen-v.$_{12}$, chin.$_{12}$, chin-s.$_{12}$, lyc.$_{12}$, op.$_{12}$, pimp.$_2$, sal-ac.$_{12}$

Figure 10
Remedies with an Action Similar to Chenopodium

Tinus Smits, MD

SACCHARUM OFFICINALE, THE MAGIC SUGAR!

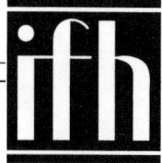

Tinus Smits has studied homeopathy for 19 years under such teachers as Jacques Imberechts, Alex Jacques, and Alfons Geukens. He practiced for ten years as a lay homeopath before starting his medical training. For the last seven years Tinus has been teaching homeopathy in several countries, using video cases and live consultations. In 1990, he published A Practical Materia Medica for the Consulting Room *(second edition, 1992). In February 1992, he published an article in* Homeopathic Links *on the mental picture of Cuprum metallicum. This article won an award from the Liga Medicorum Homoeopathica Internationalis for the best homeopathic article published in 1992. It also won a first award in the category of materia medica from the National Board of Homeopathic Examiners in the United States.*

[Editors' Note: Scattered throughout Dr. Smit's presentation are reference abbreviations for various Saccharum symptoms: TA is T.F. Allen's encyclopedia; WB is William Boericke's materia medica; Cl is J.H. Clarke's dictionary; and TS is Tinus Smits. Any spontaneous comments made by Dr. Smits are bracketed and italicized.]

Introduction: Shaking the Sugar Tree

I am quite pleased to be here. I have really enjoyed myself at this conference and in America generally. Thank you for all the beautiful cases you have shown me. As the last speaker, I will try to finish the weekend with equally good cases.

I'd like to begin by playing some music for you, as Steve Olsen did yesterday. I think it will put you in a good frame of mind to understand the remedy Saccharum.

There is a story about this song. When I was teaching in Santa Fe last year, I showed some Saccharum cases. One of the students heard a song on her car radio as she drove home from the seminar, and she thought it was a good example of the Saccharum energy. Indeed, it is. As you will see, it expresses many aspects of the remedy.

(Plays the following song.)

SHAKE THE SUGAR TREE

by Chapin Hartford

Love, you're getting lazy
You're forgettin' to give me
Sweet sugar words that I want to hear
You've been neglectin' me
You know jealousy, it is bitter as a green spring berry

You're like fruit from a fickle vine
You turn sweet in the nick of time
Love, you only come alive when you're losin' me
And it's a childish game
I've got to shake you up just to wake you up
To make you love me
I'll shake the sugar tree
Till I feel your love falling all around me
You've got to tend to what you've planted
And if you take my love for granted
baby I'll shake the sugar tree

Another night and you're sleepin'
I'm awake and I'm dreamin'
Oh honey 'bout the way you used to be
A little time's gone by
Now do you think that I'm content
With the cookin' and the payin' of the rent
No, I wanna know if your love's all spent

When I prescribed Saccharum officinale for the first time about one year ago, I didn't realize that this prescription would be the starting point for the discovery of a remedy that has now taken a very important place in my practice. It was the case of a seven-year-old boy with hay fever and problems with aggression. (See Case Number 1 later in the presentation.) The picture of this case was not at all clear for me.

I had just read about Saccharum in Clarke. My thought was that there must be Saccharum patients in our culture because we consume so much sugar each day, just as there must be Coffea and Thea patients created from our consumption of those substances. In Clarke, you will find that children are said to be very aggressive after eating sugar. So, I decided to prescribe Saccharum officinale because of his great desire for and striking aggravation from eating chocolate and sugar. And the remedy had a marvelous effect!

My second Saccharum case was really a beautiful one. (See Case Number 2 later in the presentation.) It helped me to understand the deeper mechanisms of the Saccharum patient. The patient was a 3½-year-old boy with eczema and an insatiable desire for chocolate and sweets. Within two weeks after giving him Saccharum officinale his desire had disappeared; within three months his eczema had disappeared. Most notable was the boy's reaction three days after the remedy. He woke in the middle of the night, weeping and wanting to be held tightly by his mother. This behavior continued for two nights.

I thought a lot about this second case. This boy obviously needed so much sugar and sucked his fingers because there was a strong suppressed need for affection. This real need for affection came up after the Saccharum, was satisfied, and then everything was all right. He didn't need sugar anymore after that. Sucking expresses the need for affection. The first thing we do when we are born is to suck the mother's breast. When that is not possible or when there are problems with nursing, then a Saccharum patient can easily be created.

Through my study of Saccharum officinale as a new "arrow" on the homeopathic "bow" I have become impressed by the influence of sugar on our health. Today, everyone is convinced of the adverse effects of smoking and of alcohol and drug abuse. But sugar is rarely suspected as a toxic agent, except for its relationship to obesity. Nevertheless, the great Dr. Hering warned us a century ago that a large proportion of chronic diseases in women and children are caused by the use of too much sugar (WB). Leg ulcers and myocardial degeneration were known to be caused by the use of sugar (WB).

At that time, sugar was already known for a number of uses:

- As an antiseptic, combating infection and putrifaction (WB).

- As a solvent, acting on fibrin, stimulating secretion by the intense osmotic changes induced, and thus rinsing out the wound with serum from within and favoring healing (WB).

- As a nutrient and tonic in wasting disorders, anemia, neurasthenia, and so forth, increasing weight and power (WB).

I have found Saccharum officinale to be an important remedy for all kinds of infections with foul, purulent discharges, such as sinusitis, chronic rhinitis, and otitis. Probably the excessive use of sugar in our modern society (about 130 pounds and 100 pounds per person each year in the United States and Europe, respectively) is responsible for a number of chronic infections and chronic diseases. Dr. Hering said that sugar provokes a degeneration of blood vessels resulting in bad circulation and arteriosclerosis.

Examples of Typical Saccharum Patients

In the following paragraphs, I'll describe a child and an adult who exemplify Saccharum characteristics. Clarke describes Saccharum children as overweight, resembling Calcarea, but I have found that most Saccharum children are thin and very pale. Adult Saccharum patients display much more obesity.

The Saccharum Child

Male
Age 3½

Chronic ear problems since he was ten months old.

Diminished hearing.

Chronic colds October through April with frequent epistaxis, recurrent otitis media, and an almost chronic ear discharge.

Gets tubes inserted in his eardrums every winter.

Perspires a lot, especially on his neck at night.

Profuse salivation day and night.

Mouth is always open.

Aggressive behavior; quick-tempered; spits on other children; throws things; kicks or bites other children.

Very changeable moods.

Afraid of nothing (but was afraid of water and screamed loudly when he was a baby).

Cuddles only with his mother.

Started walking when he was 1½ and started to speak early.

Warm. Wears shorts in the winter and likes to walk in bare feet.

Enormous need for sweets; accepts only soft food; very thirsty for cold drinks; loves lemons and eggs; averse to warm food and cooked vegetables; loves raw vegetables.

Plan: First, I gave him Belladonna 1MK, with some good results. The most remarkable result was the disappearance of his bad temper after waking. But the Belladonna did not produce a real breakthrough:

He continues to have ear problems from time to time

He still has a big hole in his left eardrum, and the ear, nose, and throat specialist is considering a transplant.

His character has not really changed.

He is very restless.

He still perspires a lot on the head and the neck at night.

He has to eat frequently; when playing outside, he often comes back into the house to ask for candy. He has to eat immediately when he wakes in the morning.

He became aggressive after his grandmother had given him too much candy.

He is very sensitive to pain.

He never sucks his thumb and never puts anything in his mouth.

When he has to leave home to go to scouts, he complains of nausea and pain in the abdomen.

Plan: Then, I gave him Saccharum officinale 10MK, once a month for five months. This remedy produced a dramatic change on every level.

His ear problems have disappeared completely. His left eardrum closed totally in two months.

He salivates much less.

His mouth closed gradually.

He perspires normally now.

His behavior changed dramatically. He is less restless, his temper has stabilized, and he is not aggressive anymore. He still has an abnormal need for sweets and cuddling.

Plan: I am continuing Saccharum officinale 10MK, once every two months.

The Saccharum Adult

Female
Age 55

Always hungry and has to eat every one or two hours; otherwise, trembles and feels weak.

Nauseated if eats sweets when hungry, even a little bit of chocolate is too much.

Aversion to sweets, even as a child.

Sucked her thumb until age seven, when she first got braces on her teeth.

Irritable after waking in the morning until after breakfast.

As a child, sudden fits of blind anger, very aggressive, hit and kicked others.

Sudden anger; barely able to control herself.

Homesick; difficulty in taking leave of persons and objects.

Cried last year when she exchanged her old car for a new one.

Helps others; pays too little attention to herself.

Plan: The other symptoms indicate Carcinosin without any doubt. I hesitated whether to first give Carcinosin and then Saccharum, but I decided to start immediately with Saccharum officinale 10MK.

Her feeling of hunger has changed completely.

She eats much less and doesn't feel the need to eat between meals anymore.

She is feeling much better.

She can eat sweets now without feeling nauseated.

Hypoglycemia: A Disturbed Sugar Metabolism

In my practice I have found several indications for hypoglycemia or problems related to a disturbed sugar metabolism:

- Ravenous appetite soon after eating.
- Constant appetite; never satisfied.
- Sleeplessness, ameliorated by eating.
- Tendency to eat frequently between meals.
- Irresistible desire for sweets.
- Strong impulse to eat on waking, often because of a faint feeling or weakness.
- Trembling and irritability when hungry, especially on waking.

The great material cause of hypoglycemia is without any doubt the excessive use of rapidly metabolized carbohydrates (sugar) in our modern diets.

The other material causes are the use of caffeine, alcohol, and cigarettes. The caffeine in coffee, cola, tea, chocolate, and cocoa stimulates the suprarenal glands to release adrenaline, which in turn stimulates the release of sugar from the liver into the blood. About 70 percent of alcohol abusers suffer from hypoglycemia. And the amount of sugar in the blood increases after a cigarette.

The emotional causes of hypoglycemia include lack of affection, inability to handle affection, and stress.

Hypoglycemia strongly influences our social behavior and emotional well-being. Dr. Michael Lesser stated that 67 percent of his psychiatric patients suffer from hypoglycemia. Several research studies show that our behavior becomes erratic, violent, and antisocial under the influence of hypoglycemia. And this is what I see in many of my patients with an unstable sugar metabolism, especially children. They exhibit violent fits of anger with striking, kicking, vandalism, aggression, and discontent.

Researchers discovered that the behavior of juvenile delinquents ameliorates if they are put on a sugar-free diet. One study found that 82 percent of a group of 106 juvenile delinquents suffered from hypoglycemia. And, by simply changing their diet, the social behavior of the majority changed dramatically (*Spiritual Nutrition and the Rainbow Diet* by Dr. Gabriel Cousens).

Compensatory Mechanisms for
Lack of Attention, Affection, and Love

To prescribe Saccharum officinale with success, we have to understand the two main reactions of someone who is profoundly frustrated in their need for love and affection. The person either tries to compensate for this lack or refuses any form of affection. This is the reason Saccharum has so many opposite symptoms:

- An insatiable appetite accompanied by bulimia, or no appetite at all accompanied by anorexia.
- A thirst for large quantities, or no thirst at all.
- A great need to cuddle, or refusing every contact.
- Exaggerated thumb sucking, or no thumb sucking at all.
- Sensitive to pain, or almost insensitive to pain.
- No appetite in the morning, or ravenous appetite on waking so that they have to eat immediately.

We sometimes see these kinds of contradictory symptoms in the same person. For example, the person may alternate between gentle and very aggressive behavior. Or the person may have cold feet but may sometimes put them outside the covers at night because they feel so hot.

The predilection for compensating for a lack of affection seems to be by far the most prevalent reason for the use of sweets of any kind. There is a definite link between love and sweets. That's why we talk of a "sweet" boy or girl and why we call our beloved "honey," "sweetheart," and so forth. In our twentieth-century culture, sweets play an enormous role in compensating for our deep and even superficial frustrations.

That's why the Saccharum patient displays so many symptoms in relation to food desires and aversions, to appetite and eating. The most frequent symptom is the exaggerated desire for any kind of sweets, especially for chocolate, licorice, pastries, and biscuits. The increased desire for sweets or increased appetite before menses and the desire for sweets after dinner are also strong in Saccharum.

An increase in appetite as the day progresses is typical. Frequently, we see no appetite at all in the morning after rising. The appetite increases by the afternoon and especially in the evening, with a tendency to eat candy in the evening while there is not such a need during the day.

Another group, which is more or less subject to hypoglycemia, has a strong need to eat immediately on waking and a tendency to eat frequently between meals, not feeling well if the meal is postponed a little. They feel weak, trembling, empty in the stomach, dizzy, and headache-prone if they can't eat at regular hours. They feel weak and irritable in the morning, have difficulty activating themselves, and feel generally better after breakfast.

Although Saccharum patients can exhibit a lack of appetite and thirst, an insatiable appetite and a great thirst are more common.

In children, we can see the compensatory mechanisms more clearly. They have a great need for cuddling. They suck their thumb and bite their nails (transformed to an uncontrollable need to smoke in adults), putting everything in the mouth and touching everything. I have frequently seen the relation between sucking the thumb and smoking. Many patients admitted that they exchanged the first for the latter. I was amazed to find so many adults who were still sucking their thumb. Many people smoke to reduce or to control their weight because they experienced that stopping smoking meant eating more, especially sweets.

Another compensatory mechanism is loquacity. Most patients are not aware of their secret need for attention. Children have many means at their disposal for getting attention. They can do pranks, ask again and again for something, do things that are forbidden, ask constantly for attention when their parents are talking with someone else, act jealous of their brother or sister, act restless, shout, fight, cry, have pain, become ill.

In adults, these mechanisms can persist or change into more adult-like forms, such as the exaggerated need to possess objects or to have new things, with a constant feeling of dissatisfaction. Also the incapacity to have a deep and lasting relationship with someone, looking again and again for a new love affair but never finding what they are really seeking. They are like a perforated bucket. You can put all the water you want in it, but the bucket will empty itself constantly. There is a fundamental and profound frustration from early life that cannot be satisfied. (See Case Number 2.) Only a deep transformation and cure can help such a person, and homeopathy can be a very effective tool for this.

Obesity and Weight Loss

Obesity is linked to a lack of affection. Most obese people spend their lifetime trying desperately to lose weight. The problem is that there is a profound frustration underneath the exaggerated need to eat. The body holds a deep fear of lack of affection in the future, so it transforms every ounce to fat and retains this fat. This is the way the body assures its reserves.

When obese people follow a starvation diet and lose 10 or 20 pounds they start to compensate for the frustrating diet and regain their initial weight in some months or even quicker. Only a person with a very strong will can succeed in such an enterprise. With Saccharum we can often help this type of patient more efficiently and profoundly by treating the underlying problem.

Differential Diagnosis

To me, Saccharum officinale most resembles Belladonna, Calcarea carbonica, Carcinosin, Chamomilla, Cuprum metallicum, Lachesis, Lycopodium, Opium, Stramonium, and Tuberculinum bovinum.

First, let's discuss the group of restless children with behavior problems. For this group, Saccharum officinale most resembles Belladonna, Carcinosin, Chamomilla, Cuprum metallicum, Stramonium, and Tuberculinum bovinum. In the new *Repertorium Homeopathicum Syntheticum*, edited by Dr. Frederik Schroyens, the important rubric of restless children is, in my experience, still lacking some important remedies such as

Belladonna, Cuprum metallicum, Stramonium, and, probably the most important of all, Saccharum officinale.

Belladonna shares the following symptoms with Saccharum officinale: congestion of the head; flushing; restlessness; aversion to warm food, vegetables, and milk; aggressiveness with striking and kicking; waking from fright; bed-wetting; maliciousness; irritability on waking; impulse to touch everything; changeable mood; and defiance. Both are important remedies for flushes during menopause.

The resemblance with **Calcarea carbonica** is logical, because sugar is interacting with the calcium metabolism. The common symptoms are as follows: obesity; tiredness; obstinacy; aversion to warm food; desire for sweets, ice cream, and milk; complaints before menses, including sadness, irritability, pain in mammae, swelling of mammae; head congestion; cold feet, becoming too warm in bed; perspiration of the head, especially at night; and constipation.

Chamomilla can be difficult to differentiate because of the following symptoms: violence; violent anger; kicking and striking; irritability; sensitivity to pain; extreme thirst; desire to be carried; restlessness; and profuse perspiration at night.

The differential diagnosis with **Stramonium** also can be very difficult because Saccharum officinale has almost the same forsaken feeling with the enormous anxiety at night and the fear of being alone at night, obliging the parents to stay with the child until the child falls asleep again. Other common symptoms are as follows: clinging to the mother; ceaseless talking; extreme thirst; violence and violent rage; painlessness of usually painful complaints; jealousy; restlessness; and running about.

Another important differential diagnosis to make is with **Lachesis**, which shares the following symptoms with Saccharum: loquacity; jealousy; homesickness; depression in the morning and excitement in the evening; aversion to being touched; flashes of heat during menopause; and sensitivity to pain. You can see enough common symptoms that making a choice is difficult.

The Saccharum patient can be very tense sometimes, with cramps. This can make it difficult to differentiate from **Cuprum metallicum**. The common symptoms are as follows: aversion to being touched; lassitude; sensitivity to pain; restlessness; cold feet; timidity; dictatorial behavior; amelioration from being carried about; irritability; destructiveness; night terrors; and loquacity. (See my article on Cuprum metallicum published in the February 1992 edition of *Homeopathic Links*.)

347

Lycopodium can greatly resemble Saccharum. When you are sure that you have a Lycopodium patient and the remedy doesn't work, you have a good chance that the remedy is Saccharum. I had several such cases that proved to be Saccharum. The resemblance is striking: dictatorial behavior; want of self-confidence; need of approbation; fear of undertaking new things; oversensitivity to pain; irritability and sadness in the morning on waking; desire for sweets; insatiable appetite; defiance; disobedience; insolence; unrefreshed sleep; and restlessness while sitting.

Tuberculinum bovinum has the following symptoms in common with Saccharum: alternating moods; maliciousness; aggressive and destructive behavior; irritability in the morning on waking; dissatisfaction; profuse perspiration during sleep; chronic colds; desire for sweets, salt, and milk; thirst for large quantities; ravenous appetite; restlessness, with an impulse to run; capriciousness; striking; obstinacy; anxiety at night; and bed-wetting.

It was rather surprising to me to find **Opium** as a remedy close to Saccharum. The most striking common symptoms are as follows: insensitivity to pain; irresolution; open mouth; and constipation with hard balls.

I purposely kept **Carcinosin** for the end, because it has its own history. When the picture of Saccharum became more and more clear to me I was struck by its likeness with Carcinosin. I had several cases with an almost complete picture for both Carcinosin and Saccharum. I decided not to take up the specific symptoms of Carcinosin in the picture of Saccharum, fearing that I would not be able to distinguish them later. And that was a lucky choice. Much later I understood that these remedies follow one after another, first Carcinosin and then Saccharum. This gave me the option to continue the treatment of a lot of Carcinosin patients when their case was no longer progressing.

I am still working out the relationship between Saccharum and Carcinosin, but I need more information over a longer period of time before I publish my findings. In my opinion, the main difference is that Saccharum patients compensate rather well for their need for love and affection; Carcinosin patients are much less able to do so and are much more liable to victimize themselves. But there still are a lot of questions to answer.

Finding the Optimal Dosage: Unresolved Problems

Often, after a patient takes Saccharum, rather serious aggravations appear, especially acute infections but also pain and mental disturbances. One patient said to me,

"I'll never take this horrible medicine again," after I had given her Saccharum officinale 200K. She felt very depressed and had a strong desire to commit suicide. I reconsidered her case carefully and was certain that Saccharum was her remedy. So I convinced her to take Saccharum officinale LM6 every day until she felt any aggravation. Two weeks later she telephoned. She enthusiastically told me that her depression was completely gone and that she never felt better.

Other patients get infections such as otitis, sinusitis (often), angina, bronchitis, bursitis, and panaritium. It has been difficult to resolve these problems with lower potencies of Saccharum in a solution or with more specific remedies, and sometimes I have not been able to avoid using antibiotics. I am trying to find out whether Saccharum album (rather than officinale) is a better choice in these cases.

I am still working out optimal potencies in order to avoid too severe or too long-lasting aggravations. Nevertheless, one thing is absolutely certain. Saccharum officinale is a very deep-acting remedy that touches profound mechanisms in the human being, and it can be hazardous to give the high potencies that classical homeopaths use. For adults, I often start with 30 or 200K. For children in relatively good health and with behavioral problems, I often give 10MK without any problem. I repeat the 30K every week, the 200K every two weeks, the 1MK every three weeks, and so on.

Synthesis of Saccharum Officinale

Adults and Children

1. Type: pale, death-like face (Cl); dry skin; obesity with compulsive eating, especially sweets, cakes and pastries, potato chips—anything. Very aggressive children, often emaciated.

2. FAMILY history of DIABETES and cancer.

3. AILMENTS from lack of affection; lack of physical contact in early childhood—especially babies who didn't get breast-feeding—combined with a lack of contact with the mother; lack of attention; lack of love; behavior rewarded by sweets.

4. A desperate search for love and affection because of a fundamental frustration in affection in the past, mostly in early childhood.

5. Great need to CUDDLE, to be caressed and touched, or difficulty in admitting this need and refusing every contact.

6. SUCKING THE FINGERS OR THUMB almost the whole day and during the night, or having never sucked the thumb at all. Putting everything in the mouth, or never putting anything in the mouth. Sucking the thumb until an advanced age. [*I have been surprised to discover how many adults suck their thumb or fingers. If you ask them, they will say, "Yes, sometimes when I am in bed or alone in front of the TV, I put my thumb in my mouth."*]

7. BITING NAILS, up to the quick; biting toenails. [*Smoking is the same thing. It is another oral expression, a more adult expression, of the need for love. I have often observed that heavy smokers stopped biting their nails or sucking their fingers after beginning to smoke. When they stop smoking they start to bite their nails again or they eat sweets, but it is the same. Often people smoke to control their weight, so you can see all of this is the same problem.*]

8. HOMESICKNESS (TA, TS). Difficulty in taking leave of people or objects. Difficultly in accepting losses. [*This is logical. When you feel a lack of love and affection, it is mainly with the mother. Saccharum expresses more the mother principle. Carcinosin is more the father principle—the ego, the self-confidence. Often my Carcinosin patients tell me they feel much more after taking the remedy and they no longer try to constantly please others, which is a big change. Saccharum is working much more on the mother principle—love, affection, and attention. Homesickness is a very important symptom in the Saccharum picture. There is also a tendency to have many objects around them, hence the difficulty in taking leave of people and letting go of objects. It is an attachment, an insecurity.*]

9. JEALOUSY, from fear of losing the beloved. VERY UNCERTAIN ABOUT THE LOVE OF PARTNER OR PARENTS.

10. LOQUACITY, MOSTLY TO HAVE ATTENTION.

11. IRRESOLUTION.

12. IRRITABLE (Cl), morning, until breakfast; when one or two hours without taking any food; irritable when hungry, ameliorated by eating.

13. Slow to wake up and revive after rising in the morning.

14. ALTERNATING MOODS, gentleness alternating with aggression.

15. SENSITIVE TO PAIN or NOT SENSITIVE TO PAIN AT ALL. FAINTING FROM PAIN. Fear of fainting. Fear of seeing blood. Fainting on seeing blood. Fainting from a blood puncture.

16. RESTLESS; restless legs.

17. AGGRAVATION: sweets; chocolate; warm weather; in early morning (Cl), with difficulty in starting the day.

18. AMELIORATION: evening; sweets (Cl); eating (Cl); after breakfast.

19. AVERSION: (cooked) vegetables; warm food; anything except sweets (Cl); sweets; warm milk; fat; butter.

20. DESIRES: chocolate, licorice, sweets, pastries and cakes; sweets after dinner and before menses; raw vegetables; tea; COLD DRINKS, especially water; (warm) milk; fat; salt; butter; bread and butter; sour; lemons; mustard. [*In my experience, 80 percent of Saccharum patients say they desire licorice.*]

21. THIRST for large quantities. Desires water. Or absence of thirst.

22. Ravenous appetite soon after eating with feeling of emptiness in stomach and general weakness. Tendency to eat frequently between meals. Has to eat at the normal hour, otherwise weak, dizzy, trembling, headache. Ravenous appetite, morning, after waking, has to eat first. Insatiable appetite not ameliorated by eating.

23. Little or no appetite in the morning, but insatiable appetite in the evening, especially for sweets. No feeling of hunger at all at any time; no desire to eat.

24. COMPULSIVE EATING. Bulimia with obesity.

25. WEAKNESS, lack of energy. Sudden weakness, ameliorated by eating. Weakness after sweets.

26. Extremely AGGRESSIVE, quarrelsome (Cl), violent (TA), malicious and defiant, especially after eating chocolate or sweets. Kicks and hits.

27. FITS OF ANGER, unapproachable.

28. SADNESS, aggravated after sweets. Lack of joy in life, feeling that life is not worth living. No real feeling of relationship with other people and with life in general. Feeling that everybody in the world is against him. Hypochondriacal mood (Cl).

29. Sensation of LONELINESS. FORSAKEN FEELING.

30. DISCONTENTED with himself and with everything. Hard to please.

31. TIMIDITY. FEAR OF FAILURE (Carcinosin). Sensitive to criticism; great need of approbation.

32. FEAR OF DARK. FEAR OF LOSING BELOVED PERSONS AND PARENTS.

33. FEAR OF FAILURE. WANT OF SELF-CONFIDENCE.

34. PHYSICAL TENSION.

35. WAKING VERY EARLY IN THE MORNING.

36. Instability of body temperature. Extreme chilliness alternating with heat, especially at night. Hot feet, sticks them out of bed, often only one foot. Sticks one or two arms out of bed or sleeps with the upper half of body uncovered.

37. Extreme DRYNESS: dryness of skin, hair, nails, hands, feet, inside of nose, eyes, mouth, throat, vagina, stool.

38. Painful ovulation and menses. Complaints before menses including sadness, irritability, swelling and painful breasts (Sepia, Carcinosin). Brown bloody discharge preceding menses.

Children

1. Type: very pale, white as sugar. Perspiration of the head, especially at night.

2. Great need to CUDDLE, to be caressed and touched, or difficulty in admitting this need and refusing every contact.

3. TOUCHING EVERYTHING.

4. SUCKING THUMB almost the whole day and during the night, or never sucking the thumb at all. Putting everything in the mouth, or never putting anything in the mouth; sucking the thumb until an advanced age.

5. BITING NAILS, up to the quick. Biting toenails.

6. HOMESICKNESS (TA).

7. LOQUACITY, mostly to have attention.

8. PLAYS ANTICS to have attention.

9. FORSAKEN FEELING. Desire to be held in the mother's arms. Desire to be carried.

10. ANTISOCIAL. Thinks he is neglected and placed at a disadvantage. Feels despised. Envious. JEALOUSY. VERY UNCERTAIN ABOUT THE LOVE OF PARENTS. Possessive love.

11. TIMIDITY. FEAR OF FAILURE. Sensitive to criticism. Great need of approbation.

12. SENSITIVE TO PAIN, or NOT SENSITIVE TO PAIN AT ALL. FAINTING FROM PAIN. Pain around the navel, from difficulty in letting go of the mother.

13. RESTLESS, aggravated after eating sweets; running, moving all the time. Restless while sitting. [*It is a good remedy for students who have difficulty concentrating and who eat sweets during their study time.*]

14. Fear of unknown situations (Lycopodium, Stramonium). Very uncertain.

15. Extremely AGGRESSIVE, quarrelsome (Cl), violent (TA), malicious, and defiant, especially after eating chocolate or sweets. Kicks and hits.

16. FITS OF ANGER. Unapproachable.

17. ALTERNATING MOODS, gentleness alternating with aggression.

18. WAKING EARLY IN THE MORNING.

19. Insolence (TA). Disobedience.

20. Sensitive to reprimand, or not sensitive to reprimand at all (Tuberculinum). Impossible to correct.

21. Aphthae. Profuse salivation.

22. Delusion that his parents don't love him or that he is less loved than his siblings.

23. Always cross and whining, and, if old enough, insolent and does not care to occupy himself in any way. Everything is too much trouble (Cl).

24. RESERVED. Difficult to make contact with.

Case Number 1

Male
Age 7

Initial Visit

He has hay fever with painful running eyes during spring, summer, and autumn.

Frequent epistaxis.

Is intolerant of warm weather. His eyes become painful from sunlight; wears a cap at the least sign of sunshine; becomes aggressive in warm weather.

Sneezes often.

Open mouth.

Uses an antihistamine (Triludan) without much benefit.

His behavior becomes difficult after he eats chocolate or sugar: very aggressive; sudden anger; malicious; tries to hurt his mother by breaking her favorite objects while looking at her with a malicious smile; very restless, wild, insolent, and foolish behavior.

Otherwise, he is timid and withdrawn. Not aggressive at all. Never fights with or strikes other children.

Has never sucked his thumb or put anything in his mouth.

Did not breast-feed.

Afraid of failure and the dark.

He is hard on himself; doesn't weep when he has pain.

Desires sweets, chocolate, jam, and beans.

Plan: Saccharum officinale 10MK, single dose.

Follow-Up

The first few days he was very tense; afterwards he was much more open and was not aggressive, even after eating chocolate.

He has no desire for sweets or chocolate anymore.

Not as afraid of failure, daring for the first time in his life to go out shopping for his mother.

Not as afraid of the dark.

His hay fever is gone like snow in the sun! There is no sneezing, no problems with his eyes, no bleeding nose.

Less appetite.

Mouth is closed more often.

Fourteen months later he is still fine, but needs Saccharum officinale 10MK occasionally to correct his behavior.

Case Number 2

Male
Age 3 ½

Initial Visit

He has had eczema since he was two months old on his lower abdomen, scrotum, penis, groins, and inner thighs.

He has a gentle character; cheerful and has much fantasy in his play.

Insatiable desire for sweets and chocolate.

Aversion to warm food and vegetables during his first 18 months.

Salivates a lot during the day.

Stopped breast-feeding after six weeks because of an inflammation of the mother's breast.

Sucks on a pacifier during the night.

Doesn't suck his thumb during the day.

Irritable in the morning after waking, until after eating breakfast.

Afraid of the dark.

His anterior fontanelle closed slowly.

He started walking at 18 months.

Plan: Saccharum officinale 10MK.

Follow-Up

After three days he woke up in the middle of the night, weeping sadly and wanting to sleep with his mother. He asked her to hold him tightly in her arms; every time she released him he woke up and asked her to hold him again. He repeated this behavior the following night.

Two weeks later his excessive desire for sweets was completely gone.

He is salivating less.

Doesn't need his pacifier anymore.

No irritability before breakfast.

No fear of the dark.

He started to eat vegetables.

His eczema disappeared slowly within three months.

Case Number 3

Male
Age 8

Initial Visit

He is easily disturbed. He has thin skin, both literally and figuratively.

He screams and shrieks with closed fists.

Aggressive, striking and kicking.

Weeps easily.

He reacts dramatically to pain.

Does not feel accepted or loved by his parents. "The world is against me."

Desires death.

He is a bad loser.

Discontented.

He is hard to please; always desires something else.

Weak.

Tired.

Nauseated; pain in his abdomen.

Perspires at night.

Wakes at 5 or 5:30 a.m.

Wet his bed until he was 7½.

Constipated; suffered from diarrhea until one year ago.

Allergic to sugar. When he eats sugar he starts to tease, kick, and strike others and becomes insolent. He's better with a sugar-free diet.

Desires sweets.

He eats all day. Becomes irritable if he goes two hours without eating.

Allergic to the sun.

Family history of diabetes.

He has warts on the toes of his left foot.

Plan: Saccharum officinale 10MK.

Follow-Up

He had a strong aggravation during the first two weeks:

- "Enfant terrible."
- Very sensitive, shouting.

- Very irritable before breakfast.
- Thinks he is despised and neglected.
- Doesn't accept agreements.
- Bored with everything.

Then he had a slow recovery (3½ months later):

- Calm, much more approachable even during pain and anger.
- Less aggressive.
- More socialized.
- Less weeping.
- No longer discontented.
- No night perspiration.
- No pain in the abdomen.
- No irritability after two hours without eating.
- A little less desire for sweets.

He still has the following symptoms:

- Wakes early in the morning.
- Chaotic.
- Untidy.
- Aggravation from sugar.
- Has more warts on his toes.

Case Number 4

Female
Age 50

Initial Visit

She has many problems with her mother who reproaches her for the bad education that damaged her.

She gets very ill from eating chocolate; has an intolerance for sugar.

Her mother gave her sweets when there was a problem. She ate a lot of sugar in her childhood and was very fond of chocolate, especially from her first menses on.

Suffers from chronic constipation; has used laxatives her whole life.

She has pain in her mammae during ovulation and before menses.

Plan: Saccharum officinale 10MK.

Follow-Up

For the first two months she was very constipated and then for the first time in her life she was no longer constipated and did not need laxatives.

No more pain in her mammae during ovulation and before menses.

Is no longer a victim in her dreams.

More and more she has the feeling that she is someone.

She feels the sensation of a lump in her throat that cannot be swallowed; feels tears in her eyes, but cannot cry.

Restless legs (new symptom).

Case Number 5

Female
Age 43

Initial Visit

She has been depressed for one year.

Suffers from compulsive eating; feels mentally stronger if she eats.

Uses laxatives.

She has many fears, especially of losing control and of being rejected.

As a child she was intractable; passed her youth in different children's homes.

She gets angry easily.

Plan: Carcinosin 200K, every two weeks, and then Saccharum officinale 1MK, once a month.

Follow-Up

She was better after the Carcinosin, but she had outbursts of feeling forsaken and started biting her nails as she had done in her youth.

A week after taking the Saccharum she contracted a fever with an earache that lasted for four weeks. (She hadn't had any fever for many years.)

She would get nauseated from the odor of food.

After the second dose a month later she started having outbursts of anger.

No weakness.

No desire for sweets.

No need for laxatives anymore.

A lot of childhood feelings coming back, feelings of isolation, of rejection, of mistrust, of being forsaken.

She lost about 20 pounds in two months.

Case Number 6

Female
Age 11

Initial Visit

She is very pale and thin. Her chief complaint is that she has sleeping problems.

She wakes frequently from nightmares, with icy cold face and perspiration on her nose. Dreams that she is persecuted by people, computers, or anything—and cannot escape.

She then rises and goes to her parents' bed. Ever since she was quite young, she has been sleeping with her parents and thinks it is unjust that they can sleep together and that she has to sleep alone.

Sleeps with a four-foot-high bear.

Abhors light in her bedroom because she is afraid of the shadows.

Has curtains around her bed that completely close the space around it.

Has a very strong need for cuddling, from birth on.

Is very sensitive to pain and faints from vaccinations.

Suffers a lot from anticipation concerning school tests and homework.

Panics easily and performs much less than she could because of the panic.

Often feels nauseated in the morning on rising and also in a car.

Frequently suffers from pain around her navel.

Is irritable on waking.

Drinks a lot, especially water, emptying a glass at once.

Has a compulsive craving for chocolate.

Bites her nails.

Has always had cold hands, but regularly sticks a foot out of the covers because it feels warm.

For about the last two years, she has had about 50 mollusca on the inner side of her thighs, her labia, and around her anus.

Plan: Saccharum officinale 1MK, every three weeks.

Follow-Up: Five Months Later

Her sleep is much better.

She doesn't have nightmares anymore; no dreams of persecution.

She still has some difficulty falling asleep.

Stays in her own bed.

No more curtains around her bed.

She is less irritable on waking in the morning.

No compulsive eating of chocolate anymore.

Her school performance has considerably improved. Her anticipative anxiety is almost gone, and the panic is gone.

Feels freed from a heavy burden.

The pain around her navel is gone.

She now gets headaches (three times a week). They are mostly on the left side and occur at the end of the day, with painful eyes. Better from cold applications.

All her mollusca have gone, except two.

She has stopped biting her nails.

Has straightened her posture, looking at the world with open eyes.

Allows herself to become angry (new development), whereas before she never had the courage to defend herself.

Plan: Saccharum officinale 1MK, every three weeks.

Case Number 7

Female
Age 8

Initial Visit

In the past she had many problems with swollen tonsils, otitis, "glue" ears, and diminished hearing. Calcarea phosphorica and Lycopodium helped somewhat. Lycopodium helped a lot in changing her behavior. She had received Lycopodium 1MK in repeated doses.

Now she has dry spots around her mouth and an itching nose.

She has difficulty falling asleep; afraid of falling asleep.

Afraid of new enterprises, with much anticipation.

Has difficulty taking leave of people.

Desires to read.

Is very fastidious and punctual.

Desires to arrange everything ahead of time.

Needs reassurance.

Is dictatorial with other children. The Lycopodium 10MK is having no effect; her behavior is even worse.

Aggressive with her mother; accuses everyone, and argues about everything with her mother.

Has difficulty making contact with others. She thinks that she is not liked and is very critical of other children.

She is very restless, even in bed.

She is naughty when she comes home from school.

Adores her teacher.

Has regularly occurring herpes labialis.

Is sensitive to pain.

Refuses to be cuddled, but asks for much attention. She says to her mother, "You don't love me anymore."

Feels that she is accused of everything and that her brother is always in the right.

Complains that nobody loves her.

She gets angry when her mother leaves home and when she is reprimanded.

She lies and denies every accusation.

Plan: Saccharum officinale 10MK, three doses in an eight-month period.

Follow-Up: Ten Months Later

A great change in her behavior.

She is more social, less aggressive.

No kicking anymore.

She is not isolating herself; it is easier for her to make physical contact with others.

Milder; less dictatorial.

Better contact with other children at school.

No more feeling of not being loved. Doesn't accuse her mother of not loving her.

Less restless.

No herpes labialis.

More confidence in herself.

After taking the Saccharum, eruptions (red pimples) broke out on the back of her feet and slowly spread over her whole body.

Plan: Saccharum officinale LM6, daily.

Case Number 8

Female
Age 60

Initial Visit

She has suffered all her life from obesity.

She has an irresistible desire to eat chocolate, biscuits, and cakes, especially in the evening. She cannot imagine enjoying life without smoking and eating sweets. She never has a satisfied feeling after eating and cannot stop filling her stomach.

She hates her body because of her weight and doesn't feel comfortable in company.

She sucked her thumb until she was 14 years old.

Plan: Saccharum officinale 10MK, every four weeks.

Follow-Up

She doesn't have bouts of bulimia anymore.

She is able to control herself and is losing weight, but she still has an unsatisfied feeling and could eat all the time.

On the psychological level she feels much better.

Plan: Saccharum officinale 30K, once a week.

Follow-Up: Three Months Later

She is able to eat only at mealtimes, three times a day, and doesn't feel the need to stuff herself.

She is slowly losing weight and doesn't hate her body anymore.

Before, she didn't know who she liked and who she disliked. She didn't have feelings of sympathy or antipathy. Now she knows within five minutes how she feels about someone.

Case Number 9

Female
Age 40

Initial Visit

She has two children, ages 14 and 16. She loves her job and enjoys life.

During a routine examination a year earlier, her Pap smear tested as Class II. She was very upset because she felt completely healthy and she functioned without any problem.

She is swollen around her eyes, and her eyes are somewhat protruded. Her sclerae are very blue.

She is always hungry; she has to eat frequently, every one or two hours, otherwise she starts to tremble and feels weak. When she is in a meeting for more than two hours she has to eat.

She is not overweight.

She has an aversion to sweets. She feels nauseated even after eating a little bit of chocolate, especially when she is hungry.

She sucked her thumb until she got braces at age seven.

In the morning after rising she is irritable until she eats her breakfast.

As a child she could be very angry and aggressive. Even now she has difficulty controlling herself and has bouts of sudden anger.

Her father was calm, an introvert, and not affectionate. Her mother was dictatorial, restless, and overly affectionate.

As a child she liked to be popular and knew exactly how to get other children's attention. She still enjoys the limelight and having attention directed at her.

She was very homesick as a child, and even now she can hardly take leave of persons or objects. She cried when she exchanged her old car for a new one.

Plan: Saccharum officinale 10MK, every four weeks.

Follow-Up: Two Months Later

Great change in her appetite; she feels satisfied sooner.

She eats eight slices of bread instead of twelve.

She eats less between meals and can even wait without feeling weak and without trembling.

Plan: Saccharum officinale 10MK, every four weeks for two months, and then Saccharum officinale 10MK, every six weeks for five months.

Follow-Up: Seven Months Later

While taking the remedy every four weeks, she had some difficult weeks in feeling hungry again.

Now, after taking the remedy every six weeks for about five months so far, she feels great. No hunger between the meals, and her Pap smear is Class I again.

Case Number 10

Male
Age 5½

Case History

I saw him for the first time three years ago for diarrhea after eating solid food.

Now, he has diarrhea after drinking apple juice and eating eggs, tomatoes, fruit, and sugar.

His behavior also changes after eating this kind of food. He becomes cross, rebellious, angry, and hyperactive. He has horrible fits of temper, stamping his feet on the floor, kicking, striking, and breaking things intentionally in front of his parents, especially his mother. Defiant.

Abdominal pains.

He wants to cuddle constantly with his mother and becomes exasperated when punished.

His parents can't handle him. It's a love-hate relationship.

He bites his mother and little brother with a malicious pleasure.

Destroys things with his teeth.

His gums bleed when he brushes his teeth.

He is afraid of everyone who is taller than he, but he is the first to hit.

Very loquacious; he babbles without interruption.

He keeps talking about candies.

He perspires a lot on his head, forehead, and feet, especially at night.

He gets too warm easily.

His eyes are often inflamed with green pus, from birth on. (Earlier, I gave him Belladonna for this condition without success.)

A new investigation reveals that he becomes listless about 2 to 3 p.m.

He wants to eat the whole day, very sweet foods and warm milk.

At night he is afraid of monsters; he begins to feel anxious at twilight.

He is dictatorial, tyrannical, and easily disturbed.

He constantly asks if he is nice and if he has done well.

Suffers from flatus after eating cabbage, but Lycopodium MK ameliorates this for only a short time and when repeated it has no effect. China also ameliorates for only a short time.

Another investigation reveals that his aggression is especially directed toward his mother. He kicks and strikes her, saying that she is the most awful mother he ever saw at one moment and telling her that she is the loveliest mother in the whole world at another moment.

Clearly needs affection but is awkward in asking for it.

Is egocentric, afraid of making mistakes and of not having enough or getting less affection than his siblings.

Very jealous.

Has dry skin, especially his hands.

He still sucks his thumb.

He is very fond of raw vegetables and sweets.

Plan: Saccharum officinale 1MK, every three weeks.

Follow-Up

The results are surprising.

He has become another boy, as his mother expresses it.

After the first dose, his behavior was severely aggravated. He became very rebellious, and his parents were exasperated. But after the second dose, everything changed rapidly.

He is sociable and reasonable.

No longer aggressive.

His movements are more harmonious. He is able to compete with other children in games and is no longer afraid to lose.

He helps spontaneously with cleaning up and clearing the table.

He is able to turn down offers of sweets because he knows that it has such a bad effect on his behavior.

His fear of failure is gone, and for the first time in his life he roars with laughter.

His look is no longer malicious; it is nicer now.

The bleeding of his gums has stopped completely.

He still sucks his thumb.

Suffered from worms (Oxyuris) and was given Vermox (an allopathic drug).

He picks his nose frequently.

The dry skin on his hands was gone until two weeks ago.

Plan: Continue the Saccharum officinale 1MK, every three weeks.

Case Number 11

Female
Age 3 Weeks

Initial Visit

She constantly falls asleep when she is breast-feeding. She is losing weight, as did her older sister who was hospitalized for losing too much weight.

In the evening and at night she has cramps in her bowels and cries a lot.

She has dry skin and a rather low temperature.

Much diabetes on the mother's side. The patient's four brothers and sisters have already received Saccharum officinale for behavior problems and for a sugar allergy, with important ameliorations.

Plan: Saccharum officinale 1MK.

Follow-Up

She began to breast-feed well from the moment she took the remedy, and she is gaining weight.

Her cramps have disappeared completely.

Her skin is less dry.

(The remedy has been repeated three times now.)

Summary: Another Remedy Still to Come?

I have prescribed Saccharum approximately 400 times now. I have come to understand that there are different levels of prescription. The second level of prescription, for me, is Carcinosin, and the third level, a deeper level, is Saccharum.

I was talking with Guy Kokelenberg on the airplane as we were flying here to Seattle, and we were discussing Carcinosin and Saccharum. He said to me, "Well, the remedy I am very interested in is one which, in my opinion, follows Saccharum." I let him talk, just listened, because I am myself working on a new remedy and I was very curious to know what he thought the next remedy was. He said, "It must be mother's milk." And that is, in fact, the remedy I am now studying. I had made a new remedy that I call Lac maternum, made from the milk of nine nursing mothers. I am testing it now, to see if it follows Saccharum well. It may be a remedy that goes still deeper and has to do with cosmic love. I don't know. We will see.

Barbara Newlon: What about the effect of sugar antidoting the remedy?

Smits: I had one clear case of a Saccharum child with very difficult behavior where I gave Saccharum and it didn't work. He was even worse, yet I was sure it was a Saccharum case. We stopped the sugar completely and then the case went well. Sometimes you have to stop sugar. Often when you give Saccharum the need for sugar disappears, which is logical.

Christopher Jayne: Melissa Assilem, in England, has been doing a lot of research on the Lac humanum (human milk). Have you heard of this?

Smits: Yes. I have heard about her work. Thank you.

Stephen Gordon: In what form do you give the remedy? Do you give it on milk sugar?

Smits: Yes. I give the remedy with the granules, like other remedies. No problem.

Ahmed Currim: What has been your success using this remedy with diabetic patients? Do you have many cases?

Smits: No. I don't have many diabetic patients.

Barry Marmorstein: Is this a true constitutional remedy, or is this just an intoxication that has to be cleared out before you use the real constitutional remedy?

Smits: *I believe it is a real constitutional remedy, because it is a remedy for lack of love, which I think is very constitutional. What we do in our modern society is compensate enormously with sugar, to exist in a certain equilibrium. I have seen very beautiful cures from Saccharum. There are very deep changes.*

Ahmed Currim: *If you see a picture of Carcinosin and if you see clearly that Saccharum officinale is under the surface, will you go to Saccharum officinale immediately?*

Smits: *It depends. When there is a clear picture of Carcinosin, which is often the case in adults, I start first with Carcinosin and then afterwards I give Saccharum when the Carcinosin no longer acts. In the past, I thought I saw Psorinum coming up after Carcinosin, because I saw chilliness and the desire to eat a lot, even in the night. In reality, it was Saccharum that was coming up.*

Guy Kokelenberg: *Would you talk about your way of prescribing, "horizontally" and "vertically"?*

Smits: *I always thought that we could be doing more in homeopathy. We treat patients too "allopathically." We try to get rid of the symptoms that they present. I was interested in helping people to discover more of their goal in life, to help them to have insights into why they are on earth and so on.*

So, I began to prescribe Carcinosin frequently, because in my feeling and in my experience, it often acted more deeply than other remedies. The other remedies may act very well for some time—maybe three months, five months, six months, a year—and then, when you repeat the remedy, there is no longer a reaction. I discovered that after giving a remedy, on what I call the first level, Carcinosin often came up.

There are different levels to be treated. Everything depends on how you are taking your cases. If you take the symptoms that are there at the moment your patients come to you, this is what I call the horizontal interrogation and then you give a remedy on the first level. When you interrogate deeper to see what happened in the past, why this patient has this complaint, and how it presents in his life, this is what I call a vertical interrogation and then you will find a deeper remedy. In my experience, this is often Carcinosin and Saccharum.

So, I now often prescribe Carcinosin and Saccharum. Some colleagues have accused me of prescribing too much Carcinosin. However, in my experience, it is a very deep-acting remedy that needs to be prescribed often when the first remedy that acted very well no longer gives a positive effect.

Judith Coates: *I started a 12-step program for anorexics and bulimics. They avoid sugar for long periods of time, yet I see they still have the emotional and physical symptoms that you have outlined. I am going to give talks to two groups in the next two days. After hearing your presentation, I think I will read them your notes instead!*

I also wanted to tell you that the tobacco industry is the number two user of sugar in the world. When tobacco was sold by volume, they didn't use sugar. Now that tobacco is sold by weight, they use sugar. In the tobacco curing houses, a vaporized mist sprays sugar every 30 seconds, coating the leaves. Sugar is more addictive than nicotine when inhaled, but there are no calories from it so you can smoke and not get fat. So, it is still the same craving for sugar.

Tara Nelson: *I haven't had a chance to look very closely at the remedy Chocolate but there do seem to be some similarities between Chocolate and Saccharum. Have you thought about this?*

Smits: *I just bought the proving of Chocolate yesterday. I am very interested to study it. I think there must be some similarities.*

I am also trying to determine if there is a significant difference between Saccharum officinale and Saccharum album. For patients who are not reacting very well to Saccharum officinale, I now give them album. I think the main symptoms are the same but there can be some differences. Maybe the album is working better on infections on the physical level.

Durr Elmore: *It was an excellent presentation. Thank you very much. I think a lot of us will be using this remedy. I was just wondering why you repeat the remedy every two to three weeks?*

Smits: *I know that is a hot item. For a time, I followed Vithoulkas, who says you have to wait and wait and wait, even more than one year. I did that for some years and finally I was not content with this way of treatment. I began to repeat the remedies more frequently. I have never seen a proving from repeating the remedy and there is never a break in the healing process, except when your remedy is suppressing the symptoms.*

In my opinion, the idea of not repeating too soon, as Kent and Vithoulkas both say, for fear of spoiling case is only true for incorrectly prescribed remedies. You give a remedy with a very good result but it is only suppressing symptoms, not really curing. When you repeat the remedy, you will spoil the case or, at any rate, the cure stops and the symptoms come back. However, when you give the right remedy, you can repeat it more frequently.

I have observed the effects of repeating remedies more frequently for some years. I have found that a 30K can be given every week, a 200K every two weeks, a 1M every three weeks, and a 10M every four to six weeks. In my experience, this protocol works much more effectively. More progress is made in a shorter time. I do also have cases where patients are good for one year or more after single doses of remedies, but that is not the majority of cases. In repeating a remedy more frequently, I think we have a better tool for curing the patient and for taking them to deeper levels.

Guy Kokelenberg: *I think there is a difference between Chocolate and Saccharum. Montezuma was the first to bring chocolate to us. The chocolate was a medicine that was bitter, absolutely nothing to do with sweets. It is the Swiss who added sugar and milk to it and made it sweet, but the real chocolate addicts, and I am speaking from experience (audience laughter), love dark, bitter chocolate. So, the Saccharum qualities you have described must not be related to Chocolate. There is more anxiety in the chocolate eaters.*

Smits: *I haven't differentiated it. It is probable that Saccharum patients desire more sweet chocolate.*

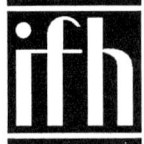